BIPOLAR DISORDER

FRANCIS MARK MONDIMORE, M.D.

Bipolar Disorder

A Guide for Patients and Families

THE JOHNS HOPKINS UNIVERSITY PRESS   BALTIMORE AND LONDON

© 1999 Francis Mark Mondimore
All rights reserved. Published 1999
Printed in the United States of America on acid-free paper
9 8 7 6 5 4 3 2

The Johns Hopkins University Press
2715 North Charles Street
Baltimore, Maryland 21218-4363
www.press.jhu.edu

Library of Congress Cataloging-in-Publication Data
will be found at the end of this book.

A catalog record for this book is available from the British Library.

ISBN 0-8018-6117-9
ISBN 0-8018-6118-7 (pbk.)

Figures 2.1, 2.4, 2.5, 5.1, 5.2, 5.4, 6.1, 10.1, 16.3, and 16.4 by Jacqueline Schaffer

Contents

Preface

About 2 percent of the population suffers from some form of bipolar disorder. Winston Churchill, George Frederick Handel, Lord Byron, Virginia Woolf, Edgar Allan Poe, Napoleon Bonaparte, and Vincent van Gogh are only a few of the politicians, writers, artists, and musicians who, despite having bipolar disorder, left a mark of greatness upon the world.[1] Most persons who are affected by this illness, however, are ordinary people who want nothing more than to get back to their everyday lives after they or their family members have been diagnosed with it. This book is written for them.

We psychiatrists have at times become a little complacent about this disease. When lithium became widely available in the United States in the mid-1970s, many psychiatrists thought that the battle to control the illness had been won. Indeed, lithium was—and still is—a miracle drug for many of those who suffer from what was then known as "manic-depression." More recent studies, however, indicate that a substantial proportion of patients have a relapse of their illness despite taking lithium—according to some studies,[2] as many as half. But even as we become more aware of the sobering facts about the difficulty of successfully treating this illness, an explosion of developments in science and medicine is occurring that holds great promise for those affected by the disease. In this book I shall relate this good news.

Clinical research has shown again and again that many relapses of bipolar disorder occur not because of medication failure, but rather because patients stop taking medication and drop out of treatment. Perhaps patients don't understand that relapse and repetition of illness episodes are the hallmark of the illness, that *abruptly* stopping medication has been shown to be especially risky, that medication side effects can often be treated or controlled, and that new medications are becoming available all the time. I hope this book helps those who face difficult treatment decisions to make well-informed and intelligent choices.

A survey of patients with bipolar disorder and other mood disorders done by the National Depressive and Manic-Depressive Association in the early 1990s found that 36 percent of those who responded to the questionnaire did not seek professional treatment until more than *ten years* after their symptoms began.[3] Seventy-three percent of the bipolar patients in this study had received at least one incorrect diagnosis before being identified as having bipolar disorder—often many years after they had first sought help. The average respondent had seen 3.3 physicians before being correctly diagnosed. Why is this illness so difficult to identify correctly? One reason is that full-blown manic-depressive illness is only one of the several forms this chameleon disorder can take—and may in fact be less common than the milder forms (the so-called soft bipolar disorders). We are realizing that many patients with these milder forms of the disorder benefit from treatment with mood-stabilizing medications, too. But they can do so only if treatment is sought and the correct diagnosis is made. We shall see why many patients who have a bipolar disorder are labeled "neurotic" or receive a diagnosis of a "personality disorder." Another purpose of this book is to spread the word that symptoms of mild depression and subtle "mood swings" may be the only manifestations of a mild form of bipolar disorder that can be effectively treated.

Like any other serious illness, bipolar disorder affects not only the person who suffers from the disease but family, friends, and colleagues as well. Family support is crucial to the effective management of symptoms. The disrupted relationships and interpersonal conflicts that the symptoms of the illness can cause make bipolar disorder all the more difficult and complicated to treat. Information and understanding are part of the treatment for this disease too, and this book was written not only with the patient in mind but for his or her family and friends as well.

Bipolar disorder can be a fatal disease. Although the figures vary among studies, about 15 percent of persons with bipolar disorder commit suicide;[4] many more make suicide attempts. These are preventable deaths, because very effective treatments for this illness exist. I hope that the information this book provides about the treatment of bipolar disorder addresses some of the reasons why individuals are reluctant to enter treatment and dissuades some from stopping treatment against medical advice. Yes, it is my hope that this book will save lives.

Acknowledgments

I wish to thank those who have contributed to this project. Thanks to Robert Bright, M.D., Charles Casat, M.D., Rhonda Crow, Caroline Gretick, Sallie Mink of the Depression and Related Affective Disorders Association (DRADA) at Johns Hopkins, and Jenny Rosenthal of the Public Library of Charlotte and Mecklenburg County, who reviewed the manuscript and provided valuable feedback and much-needed encouragement.

Thanks to Jacqueline Schaffer for her handsome illustrations and to the staff of the Alan Mason Chesney Medical Archives at Johns Hopkins for the portrait of Dr. Adolf Meyer.

Special thanks to all the talented and dedicated staff of the Johns Hopkins University Press, who have been such a pleasure to work with on this as well as on my previous projects. *Thanks* is a flimsy word indeed to express my sincere and deep appreciation for the editorial skills and constant encouragement of my editor, Jacqueline Wehmueller.

Thanks, as well, to Jay Allen Rubin for countless cups of tea and for putting up with so many hours of a closed office door at home.

PART I

SYMPTOMS, SYNDROMES, AND DIAGNOSIS

A former professor of mine once told me, "When you can't figure out *what* the patient has, he or she probably has bipolar disorder." I remember thinking at the time that this was one of the most foolish things I had ever heard a Johns Hopkins faculty member say. But over the years I have come to realize that he was right (and also to realize that you don't get appointed to the faculty at Johns Hopkins by saying foolish things).

Bipolar disorder is the chameleon of psychiatric disorders, changing its symptom presentation from one patient to the next, and from one episode to the next even in the same patient. It is a phantom that can sneak up on its victim cloaked in the darkness of melancholy but then disappear for years at a time—only to return in the resplendent but fiery robes of mania. Although both depression and mania had been described over two millennia previously by Greek and Persian physicians—several of whom thought that the conditions were linked in some way—it wasn't until the early part of the twentieth century that a German psychiatrist, Emil Kraepelin, convincingly presented the idea that these opposite conditions were two sides of one pathological coin, the two profiles of a Janus-faced disease that he called manic-depressive insanity.

Why did it take over two thousand years for someone to solve a puzzle with only two pieces? Because, as my professor knew, there are so many more than two pieces to this mysterious disorder. The depressed phase can be merely gloomy or profoundly despairing; torpid and lethargic, or agitated and churning. The manic phase can be no more than a enthusiastic glow, or it can be an exultant, transcendental fervor, frenzied panic, or delirious, crashing, raving psychosis. Sometimes opposite moods seem to be combined, as inseparable as smoke and fire, mood states that have been given names like *depressive mania, manic stupor, agitated depression,* and more recently and more simply *mixed affective states.* The tendency of the illness to hibernate—for symptoms to spontaneously disappear for years, even decades at a time—adds to the confusion, perplexing the diagnostician and lulling the patient into dangerous complacency regarding the need for treatment.

In this first part, then, there are four chapters examining the symptoms, the syndromes, and the diagnosis of bipolar disorder. In chapter 1, "Normal and Abnormal Mood," we review the many symptoms of bipolar disorder, collected into three main clusters: *mania, depression,* and the *mixed mood states.* I have not minimized the severity of the symptoms in this chapter; I present all the possible symptoms of the illness, many of them frightening and terrible. But it is important to remember that not every person with bipolar disorder develops all the possible symptoms, and also that modern treatments usually prevent the development of the worst of them, many of which are now rarely seen even by psychiatrists.

In chapter 2, "The Diagnosis of Bipolar Disorder," I discuss the different forms the disorder can take. The diagnosis of bipolar disorder is complex, and there is still some disagreement about how the different symptom clusters are related to one another. Are there several different diseases of mood with different causes? Is there a group of disorders that share common features *and* common causes? Are these illness forms essentially the *same* disorder differing only in details of expression? Do these different forms remain the same over time in each patient, or can one form develop into another? The answers to many of these questions remain unknown. Nevertheless, there are several forms of the illness that can be reliably identified and separated from one another. Identifying one or another of these forms allows for predictions about the course of the illness over time and about the type of treatment that has the best chance of being effective.

In chapter 3, "A Summary of the Diagnostic Categories of Bipolar Disorder in *DSM-IV,*" I review the official classification system of the illness that is currently used by the American Psychiatric Association (and by many psychiatrists in the rest of the world). This chapter might be considered optional reading and will probably be of more interest to students and professionals concerned with the details of illness classification and diagnostic categories.

In chapter 4, "The Mood Disease," I show how psychiatrists came to realize that bipolar disorder is indeed a disease. For decades, persons afflicted with mood disorders were often given the covert message by their physicians that they themselves were to blame for their symptoms. Depression and other mood symptoms were blamed on emotional immaturity or "maladjustment" rather than being recognized as expressions of disordered functioning of the brain. It was only with the discovery of effective pharmaceuticals that psychiatry realized that bipolar disorder is indeed a disease—as real as diabetes or hyperthyroidism.

CHAPTER 1

Normal and Abnormal Mood

BIPOLAR DISORDER IS A *MOOD* DISORDER, ONE OF SEVERAL EMOTIONAL disorders whose main symptom is an abnormality of mood. The first step in understanding the illness, then, is to understand what we mean by the word *mood*. Perhaps more to the point, I want to talk about what *psychiatrists* mean by the word. The dictionary isn't much help here; it defines *mood* simply as "a conscious state of mind or predominant feeling."[1] The "predominant feeling" part of this definition begins to capture the psychiatric concept, but mood is much more than just a feeling.

Our mood includes our happiness or sadness, our state of optimism or pessimism, our feelings of contentedness or dissatisfaction with our situation, and even physical feelings such as how fatigued or robust we feel. Mood is like our emotional temperature, a set of feelings that expresses our sense of emotional comfort or discomfort.

When individuals are in a good mood, they are confident and optimistic, relaxed and friendly, patient, interested, content. The word *happy* captures part of it, but good mood includes a lot more. People in a good mood usually feel energetic and have a sense of physical well-being; they sleep soundly and eat heartily. It's easy for them to be sociable and affectionate. The future looks bright and the moment ripe for starting new projects. When we're in a good mood, the world seems a wonderful place to live in; it feels good to be alive.

When we're in a low mood, an opposite set of feelings takes over. We tend to turn inward and may seem preoccupied or distracted by our thoughts. The word *sad* captures some of the experience, but low mood is a bit more complicated. There may be a sense of emptiness and loss. It's difficult to think about the future very much, and when one does, it's hard not to be pessimistic or even intimidated by it. We may lose our temper more easily and then feel guilty about having done so. It's difficult to be affectionate or sociable, so we avoid others and prefer to be alone. Energy is low. Self-doubt takes over; we become preoccupied, worrying about how other people see us.

Abnormal Mood

Some of life's more common stresses and the normal human reactions to them are such common experiences that common terms have been coined for some mood changes—and most people recognize these mood changes as quite normal. Moving to a new community where we don't know anyone often leads to a sense of dislocation and loneliness that we know as homesickness, an unpleasant experience that may last for days or even weeks and that everyone has probably experienced at one time or another. When someone close to us dies, a profound sense of sadness and loss occurs that can become temporarily incapacitating—the deep sorrow that we call bereavement or mourning. At the time of various milestones of personal achievement, we experience changes of mood in the other direction. On the occasion of a graduation or wedding or the birth of a child, a person can be filled with joy and pride and a sense of limitless optimism that can be nearly overwhelming. We wouldn't call any of these moods "abnormal," even though they may be extreme.

Like many other things we can measure in human beings—body temperature, blood pressure, or hormone levels, for example—a person's mood state normally varies within a certain range. People are not in the same mood state all the time; it is quite normal for everyone to have ups and downs of mood. Do persons with bipolar disorder simply have higher ups and deeper downs? Well, it's certainly true that the bipolar patient's ups and downs are sometimes so far outside the range of normal that it doesn't take a psychiatrist to know that something is very wrong. But to say that persons with bipolar disorder simply have more extreme ups and downs of mood isn't quite right. Rather, the symptoms of bipolar disorder seem to be caused by a defect in the brain's *regulation* of mood.

Laura is a forty-year-old vice-president of one of the largest banks in the country.[2] When I walked out into the waiting room to call her for our first appointment, she was sitting with a lap-top computer balanced on her knees and a cellular telephone held up to her ear. "No, Steve, that's not good enough," she was saying into the phone as she nodded to me. "No, that won't work either, we need the last quarter's *real* numbers, not an estimate. Listen, I'm . . . ah . . . in the doctor's office. I'll call you in an hour." I raised my eyebrows and shook my head. "Make that two hours. Bye." Click, click, snap, the LEDs went dark, phone and computer were shut, and in a moment we were sitting in an interviewing room.

"I made this appointment as soon as I could after I read this." Laura handed me a pamphlet called *A Guide to Depressive and Manic-Depressive Illness.* The local chapter of the National Depressive and Manic-Depressive Association had been handing them out at a local shopping mall during a health fair recently. "I've known for years that something was wrong, but I didn't know what. Reading this has made me think medication might help."

"What have you noticed that's 'wrong,' as you put it?" I asked.

"I go into these, these *things,*" she started. "I get this wired, can't-slow-down feeling. I've always called it 'the crazies,' and I usually crash after it's over. Sometimes I can't get out of bed for days."

"You seem to have a very high stress job," I offered. "Maybe that's part of the problem."

"You sound like my mother. 'You don't have to take *every* promotion they offer you,' she says. But this isn't just stress, there's something else going on. The worst part is, I think these things are getting worse."

Laura's use of phrases like "the crazies" and "these things" seemed to indicate that she felt that these feelings were foreign, not like her normal feelings.

"Are you saying that sometimes your feelings and moods are controlling you rather than the other way around?" I asked.

Laura sat up straight in her chair. "That's the best way I could possibly describe it," she said decisively. "I can *feel* them coming on; it's almost physical. But I know they're . . . well, *mental,* I guess, is the best way to put it." Her face suddenly clouded over. "Does this mean I'm mentally ill?"

"Well," I said, "we know that there are illnesses that affect mood, and mood is certainly a mental state. But we have a lot more to talk about before I'll be able to say just what explains your 'crazies' the best."

Laura looked slightly relieved and said, "Well, that's why I'm here, for an explanation." She picked the brochure up from the edge of the desk. "This is the best explanation I've come across yet," she said thoughtfully. "And that means I can get rid of them, right? There's a treatment that will get rid of them?"

"There are many treatments for mood disorders. It may just take some time to find the one that works best."

"Then I came to the right place," she said as she sat back in her chair again. " 'You're not crazy,' my mother said. 'You don't need to see a psychiatrist.' "

"Well, I think your mother was at least half right." I said.

Laura smiled for the first time. "OK, then let's—" Suddenly a beep-beep-beep sounded from her jacket pocket. She took out her cellular phone again. I started to get up. "If that's, um, confidential," I offered, "I can—"

Laura pushed a button, and the beeping stopped. She put the phone back in her pocket. "No, that can't possibly be as important as this. It can wait. I want to give you my undivided attention."

"Excellent!" I thought to myself. "This is a woman who understands priorities."

Imagine a person whose body temperature regulation system doesn't work correctly—a person who suddenly starts shivering on a warm sunny day or breaks out into a sweat in a room in which everyone else is chilly. This person's reactions to warm and cold are abnormal; his or her body "thinks" it is cold when it isn't, he or she feels hot when the temperature is cool. We can think of mood disorders as problems with *emotional* temperature regulation.

In mood disorders, the mood becomes disconnected from the individual's environment, and feelings of "happy" and "sad" take on rhythms and fluctuations of their own. Sometimes the fluctuations are mild, and the affected person only seems to have *more* ups and downs than other people have and to have mood fluctuations that are more difficult to understand. But because they don't get profoundly depressed or irrationally "high," their problems are dismissed as being due to a difficult personality or "immaturity." Sometimes, on the other hand, the mood states are so extremely abnormal that a person's ability to judge reality is shattered; behavior can be bizarre and frightening. (It is in some of these cases that a diagnosis of schizophrenia can be mistakenly made in an individual and proper treatment go wanting.) If the mood-disorder patient and his or her situation are examined with enough care, however, the basic underlying problem will be found: a problem with regulation of mood.

Since the basic problem in bipolar disorder is one of *regulation* of mood, the disorder can present different symptoms at different times. Persons afflicted with the classic form of the illness have periods of severe *depression* as well as periods of *mania* (a mood state that is in some ways the opposite of depression). The observation that these two mood states both occur at various times during the course of the illness gave rise to the older name for the disorder: manic-depressive illness. Both of these opposites of mood occur in affected persons because the brain mechanisms that normally regulate mood don't work properly. This observation—that the mood states of affected persons move to either of the two polar opposite extremes of mood—gives the disorder its modern name: bipolar disorder. In the following sections we'll take a closer look at these opposites, or poles, of bipolar disorder: the manic state and the depressed state, as well as an abnormal mood state in which the two opposites seem to be combined, a condition simply called a *mixed mood state*. After becoming familiar with these mood syndromes, we shall be able, in chapter 2, to see how their various combinations define the different forms of bipolar disorder.

A word you will frequently come across in discussions of mood disorders is *affect* (pronounced with the accent on the first syllable). To be precise, *affect* refers to the appearance of a person's mood state. *Mood* refers to the patient's inner experience, while *affect* refers to what others observe about a person's mood, the external signs of mood. (Psychiatrists talk of a patient's affect being depressed or irritable and so forth.) But for our purposes, *affect* can be considered a synonym for *mood*. (The mood disorders were at one time called *affective disorders*.)

The Manic Syndrome

The manic state, or more simply *mania*,[3] is the most extreme and dramatic of the symptom clusters of bipolar disorder. Many persons who have some of the forms of bipolar disorder never have a full-blown manic episode. But since mania is the most unmistakable and probably the most dangerous of the abnormal mood states associated with mood disorders, it is a good place to start.

In the manic state, the mood regulator switches into "high." Mania usually starts gradually and may take weeks to develop fully. Although the symptoms may be almost imperceptible at first, they gradually become more extreme, more unpleasant, and more unmistakably pathological.

In the early stages of mania, the mood state of affected persons begins gradually to move "upward," and they find themselves filled with pleasant feelings of exuberance—what a physician writing almost a hundred years ago called "a welling up of a sense of well being and an overflowing of the spirits."[4] This heightened sense of well-being and confidence grows and expands and gradually evolves into euphoria. One bipolar patient described it this way:

> The world was filled with pleasure and promise; I felt great. Not just great, I felt *really* great. I felt I could do anything, that no task was too difficult. My mind seemed clear, fabulously focused, and able to make

TABLE 1-1 Symptoms of Mania

Mood Symptoms	Bodily Symptoms
Elated, euphoric mood	Increased energy level
Irritable mood	Decreased need for sleep
Grandiosity	Erratic appetite
	Increased libido
Cognitive (Thinking) Symptoms	
Feelings of heightened concentration	Symptoms of Psychosis
Accelerated thinking ("racing thoughts")	Grandiose delusions
	Hallucinations

intuitive mathematical leaps that had up to that point entirely eluded me . . . not only did everything make perfect sense, but it all began to fit into a marvelous kind of cosmic relatedness.[5]

And here we confront one of the many ironies of this illness: at the onset of an episode of the disorder, it not uncommon to feel *better* than usual. As one manic patient said, "If I'm ill, this is the most wonderful illness I've ever had."[6]

Changes in thinking accompany the changes in mood. The feeling that one is thinking more clearly and more rationally than usual is especially common in the early stages of mania. This is an especially troublesome symptom, since such a mental state hardly makes a person suspect that something is wrong. Not only does thinking seem clearer than usual to the manic patient, but a feeling that mental processes are moving *faster* than usual also develops. As with the mood changes, there is often a very gradual onset to these alterations in thinking. At first there may be only a pleasant sense of nimbleness of thinking. Invariably, however, thinking processes accelerate: "quick" becomes "fast" and finally "racing." A vivid description of this acceleration of thinking—illustrating what psychiatrists call *flight of ideas*—comes from a collection of patient accounts written early in the twentieth century:

My thoughts ran with lightning-like rapidity from one subject to another. All the problems of the universe came crowding into my mind, demanding instant discussion and solution—mental telepathy, hypnotism, wireless, telegraphy, Christian science, women's rights, and all the problems of medical science, religion and politics.

Thoughts chased one another through my mind with lightning rapidity. I felt like a person driving a wild horse at a weak rein, who dares not use force but run[s] his course, following the line of least resistance, mad impulses rush through my brain carrying me first in one direction then in another.[7]

Racing thoughts are a symptom so typical of mania that the diagnosis becomes doubtful if this symptom is absent. This tumbling, jumbled jumping from one thought to another becomes progressively worse and more unpleasant as the episode develops.

As the manic individual's thinking speeds up, his or her speech does as well. Rapid or *pressured* speech (the term normally used by psychiatrists), like racing thoughts, is nearly always seen in mania. Manic individuals speak more and more quickly as the episode develops, attempting to express the ideas that are whirling through their consciousness at ever faster speeds. A psychiatric text from the beginning of the twentieth century mentions one early researcher who actually counted the number of syllables per minute spoken by manic patients. He found that manic patients spoke 180 to 200 syllables per minute, compared with 122 to 150 syllables per minute in nonmanic persons.[8]

Sometimes the racing thoughts and pressured speech lead to an outpouring of frenzied writing:

I made notes of everything that happened, day and night. I made symbolic scrapbooks whose meaning only I could decipher. I wrote a fairy tale . . . I noted down cryptically all that was said or done around me at the time, with special reference to relevant news bulletins and to jokes which were broadcast in radio programs. The time, correct to the nearest minute, was written in the margin. It was all vitally important. [I was convinced that] the major work [that] would be based on this material would be accurate, original, provocative and of profound significance.[9]

The feelings of exuberance and overconfidence that characterize mania can lead to several patterns of behavior typical of the manic state: spending sprees, sexual promiscuity, and overuse of alcohol and other intoxicating substances.

Spending sprees can be extravagant and financially catastrophic, because the manic person has no concern for where the money will come from when the bills come due. The increased sexual feelings of this stage of mania may lead to infatuations and even betrothals. One early psychiatric expert noted that "incomprehensible engagements, also pregnancies, are not rare in these states. I know cases in which the commencement of [mania] was repeatedly announced by a sudden engagement."[10] The lack of inhibitions typical in mania may also lead to promiscuity as well as to uncharacteristic bisexual or homosexual behaviors in some persons, perhaps by "releasing" suppressed feelings.

We shall explore the complex relationship between bipolar disorder and substance abuse in chapter 15. Suffice it to say here that increased and uncharacteristic use of intoxicating substances is frequently seen in mania.

One way to understand this hedonistic triad of mania—spending sprees, sexual overactivity, and increased substance abuse—is to group these behaviors together as expressions of an increase in "motivated behaviors" seen in mania,[11] an exaggeration of the normal drives toward pleasurable goals.

There are almost always changes in sleeping and eating habits in mania. Decreased need for sleep is in fact one of the first symptoms to develop in mania—often a clue for individuals who have been manic before that another episode may be starting. Food intake is usually reduced because manic individuals simply don't have time to eat. Constantly distracted by new thoughts and ideas they feel pressed to act on, they just can't sit still long enough to finish a meal. The ensuing weight loss can be dramatic.

As the combination of euphoric mood and mental quickness develops, the manic individual begins to feel tremendously self-confident, even fearless. This is the so-called *grandiosity* of the manic state. Fears of unpleasant consequences disappear altogether, and reckless enthusiasm takes over. The affected person may seek out new adventures and experiences with no regard for the possible adverse repercussions. This is one of the points at which the manic person can begin to lose touch with reality—when the grandiose thinking leads the individual to start *believing* the great things he or she feels capable of.

In a landmark work on bipolar disorder that we'll discuss in detail in chapter 4, the German psychiatrist Emil Kraepelin recorded the symptoms and course of the illness he called *manic-depressive insanity.* (I quote Kraepelin extensively here and in the following chapter. Not only did Kraepelin write some of the most vivid and enduring descriptions of the symptoms of bipolar disorder ever written, but his insights into the different forms and the course of the illness have proven to be correct again and again.) Kraepelin's description of the grandiose delusions of mania, written in 1896, is classic:

> The patient asserts that he is descended from a noble family. That he is a gentleman; he calls himself a genius, the Emperor William, the Emperor of Russia, Christ, he can drive out the devil. A patient suddenly cried out on the street that he was the Lord God, the devil had left him. Female patients possess eighty genuine diamonds, are leading singers, leading violinists, Queen of Bavaria, Maid of Orleans, a fairy; they are pregnant, are going to be engaged to St. Francis, are to give birth to the redeemer . . . the Messiah.[12]

Modern patients are more likely to become convinced that they are president or prime minister rather than king or queen, a rock star rather than a great violinist, but the feelings that lead to such beliefs are the same: a fantastic, indescribable feeling of mental power and significance. Feelings of religious inspiration are very common. Patients may feel that they are a modern prophet, the founder of a new religion, a reincarnation of Christ, even a new god.

The "feeling good" stage of mania is sometimes very short-lived, and the elated mood and grandiosity can be quickly replaced by angry, irritable mood. Quoting Kraepelin again:

> The patient is dissatisfied, intolerant, faultfinding . . . even rough. Trifling external occasions may bring about extremely violent outbursts of rage. In his fury, he thrashes his wife and children, threatens to smash everything to smithereens . . .
>
> . . . At the most trifling affront it may come to outbursts of rage of extraordinary violence . . . clamorous abuse and bellowing, to dangerous threats with shooting and stabbing, to blind destruction and actual attacks.[13]

Sometimes the manic individual alternates quickly between elation and irritability for a time, but usually an irritable, unpleasant mood becomes predominant. It is often this irritability that brings the patient to medical attention.

As the manic state continues to develop, pressured, racing thoughts, increased energy level, and loss of inhibitions lead to more grossly disorganized and disturbed thinking and behavior. A psychiatric textbook written in the 1950s described this stage as follows:

> Driven by greater pressure of activity, terror and excitement, [the manic person] becomes violent, attacks his neighbor, begins to shout all kinds of accusations against his alleged persecutors . . . Distortions [and] misinterpretations . . . are now elaborated into delusions of persecution accompanied by violence and panic, the patient runs down the street nude, sets fire to the house, starts an argument with the police, shoots a gun on the street or starts suddenly to preach the gospel in a frenzied manner . . . If crossed or interfered with in any way he becomes abusive, destructive, homicidal.[14]

Thinking patterns not only spin faster and faster but also become more bizarre. Hallucinations can develop, and beliefs called *delusions* can occur. The very best modern written descriptions of the symptoms of severe mania are those of Kay Redfield Jamison. Dr. Jamison's nearly unique qualification to set them down is that she is an internationally recognized medical expert on bipolar disorder who suffers from it herself. This passage by Dr. Jamison is what I give medical students to read so that they can learn about the symptoms of severe mania:

> Although I had been building up to this for weeks and certainly knew something was seriously wrong, there was still a definite point when I knew I was insane. My thoughts were so fast that I couldn't remember the beginning of a sentence halfway through. Fragments of ideas, im-

ages, sentences, raced around and around in my mind like the tigers in a children's story. Finally, like those tigers, they became meaningless melted pools. Nothing familiar to me was familiar. I wanted desperately to slow down but could not. I felt my mind encased by black lines of light that were terrifying to me. My delusions centered on the slow painful deaths of all the green plants in the world—vine by vine, stem by stem, leaf by leaf they died, and I could do nothing to save them. Their screams were cacophonous. Increasingly, all my images were black and decaying.[15]

These passages vividly make the point that the manic state is not pleasant— even if it may sometimes start out that way. Those unfamiliar with the illness sometimes think that persons with bipolar disorder simply experience swings of mood between "happy" and "sad." As the foregoing illustrates, this is not usually true. The full-blown manic state is not only intensely unpleasant but also very dangerous. The danger arises not only from the increased risk of violence toward others (or toward self) but also from the physical stress the syndrome causes.

The combination of severe manic symptoms and the physical stress from such frenzied hyperactivity can lead to what Kraepelin called *delirious mania* in which there is "profound clouding of consciousness and extraordinary and confused hallucinations . . . The patients become stupefied, confused, bewildered and completely lose orientation for time and place."[16] Fortunately it is now rare for a psychiatrist to see patients suffering from this severest form of the manic state, but in Kraepelin's time and even more recently, mania had a significant mortality rate. Persons with mania died "in a state of progressive exhaustion,"[17] suffering dehydration and cardiovascular collapse.

In 1973, just as lithium, the first effective treatment for bipolar disorder, was becoming available, a study from the National Institutes of Health attempted to describe a typical manic episode from beginning to end.[18] Patients who had been admitted to a research unit that was trying to figure out how to use lithium safely and effectively for the treatment of bipolar disorder were carefully observed. The course of their symptoms was meticulously documented and described. The authors concluded that three stages could be described in a manic episode:

[Stage I]: Increased psychomotor activity which included increased . . . rate of speech and increased physical activity . . . Euphoria predominated, although irritability became obvious when the patients' many demands were not instantly satisfied . . . Expansiveness, grandiosity and overconfidence. Thoughts were coherent though sometimes [disconnected]. Also frequently observed during this stage were increased sexuality or sexual preoccupations, increased interest in religion, increased and inappropriate spending of money, increased smoking, telephone use and letter writing. Some of the patients were aware of the mood change on some level and described the feeling of "going high," having racing thoughts and feeling like they were in an airplane. At this stage the patients were not out of control.

[Stage II]: Pressure of speech and . . . activity increased still further. Mood, although euphoric at times, was now more prominently characterized by increasing [unpleasantness] and depression. The irritability observed initially had progressed to open hostility and anger, and the accompanying behavior was frequently assaultive. Racing thoughts progressed to . . . increasing disorganization. Preoccupations that were present earlier became more intense with earlier . . . grandiose trends now apparent as frank delusions.

[Stage III]: A desperate, panic stricken, hopeless state experienced by the patient as clearly [unpleasant], accompanied by frenzied and frequently even more bizarre . . . activity. Thought processes that earlier had been only difficult to follow now became incoherent . . . Delusions were bizarre . . . hallucinations were present [in about one-third of the patients].

More recently some researchers have questioned whether or not typical manic episodes include all of these stages. Specifically, some researchers believe that stage III mania (or *dysphoric mania,* as it has come to be called) occurs only in a subgroup of patients with bipolar disorder. There is some evidence that these patients have a variant of the disorder and may need medications different from what others with more typical bipolar disorder would need. (More on this in "Mixed Mood States," later in this chapter.) Nevertheless, this study on the "stages of mania" was important because its investigators used modern clinical methods to document just how very sick patients with mania can get. Even more important, it made the researchers realize that it would be easy to misdiagnose a very disorganized patient in stage III mania as having schizophrenia, a psychiatric illness that requires a very different treatment approach and has a very different prognosis from bipolar disorder.

The Hypomanic Syndrome

In 1881 a German psychiatrist named Mendel published a book about the manic state called *Die Manie* and in it proposed that another term be used for states of mild euphoria and hyperactivity that did not progress to full-blown mania. He called this condition *hypomania,* "similar to the state of exultation in typical mania [but] with a certain lesser grade of development."[19] (The prefix *hypo-* comes from a Greek word meaning "under.") Hypomania can best be thought of as consisting of the symptoms that are present at the beginning of a manic episode (stage I in the study described above): the elated mood, the increased energy level, the rapid thinking and speaking, and sometimes a bit of the irritability. Norman Endler, another psychologist who himself suffered from a mood disorder and wrote of his experiences with the illness, described hypomania this way:

> Most of the time I was busy, busy, busy; taping records, playing tennis, skiing, writing manuscripts, talking . . . reading, going to movies, staying up at night, waking up early in the morning, always on the go— busy, busy, busy. Furthermore, I was boasting about all the energy I had that enabled me to keep up this fast pace . . . Instead of occasionally "idling" in neutral I was always in overdrive.[20]

Although persons in the hypomanic stage do not have the severe mental disorganization of mania and are by definition not agitated and frenzied to the point of violence toward themselves or others, hypomania can nevertheless have unpleasant consequences. Feelings of increased confidence can lead to foolish investments in real estate or the stock market, and patients can squander personal resources on grandiose and risky business ventures. Increased sexual feelings can lead to extramarital affairs or promiscuity—actions that can be life-threatening in the age of HIV disease. The irritability of hypomania can lead to arguments and disagreements with family, colleagues, or neighbors that can sour relationships, sometimes irreparably. Dr. Endler described it this way:

> As a hypomanic, I didn't stop to analyze my thoughts, feelings, or behavior. I was much too busy and didn't always stop to think about what I was doing . . . I was critical of others and occasionally told some people off publicly. I was not so concerned about . . . the effect my behavior had on [others]. I was aggressive, talked incessantly, and interrupted others while they were speaking. Whenever I had a thought I felt compelled to utter it, and I didn't always censor my thoughts and feelings. At times I seemed to have lost my sense of judgment. I was having a good time, I was narcissistically preoccupied with myself, but (without being aware of it) I was making my wife miserable.[21]

Persons with even mild hypomania can quit a good job in a burst of overconfidence or irritability, withdraw a life's savings for a get-rich-quick scheme, or simply begin to drive their car too fast—all behaviors with potentially devastating consequences.

TABLE 1-2 Length of Time before Hospitalization in Ninety-four Manic Patients

Time	Percentage of Patients	
	Male	Female
14–30 days	69	62
3 months	11	11
6 months	11	10
1 year or more	6	15

Source: Data from George Winoker, Mania and Depression: A Classification of Syndrome and Disease (Baltimore: Johns Hopkins University Press, 1991), 13.

Note: Notice that some patients have symptoms for many months before receiving needed treatment. During this time, hypomanic symptoms can wreak havoc on their lives.

Words like *seductive* and *addictive* are frequently applied to the hypomanic syndrome. Because individuals in a hypomanic state feel so good, they seldom seek treatment. Even for persons who have a history of previous manic or depressive episodes of bipolar disorder and perhaps should know that trouble is brewing, the giddy delight of being hypomanic often seems too delicious to interrupt. Persons whose abnormal mood states are successfully controlled with medication sometimes stop treatment to recapture the wonderful feelings that accompany hypomania. I have even heard fellow psychiatrists comment that it seems a shame to start medication on hypomanic persons who are "having so much fun."

Because hypomanic individuals are *not* psychotic, they often cannot be involuntarily treated for their illness because criteria for involuntary treatment insist upon "dangerous" behaviors. (We shall discuss involuntary treatment in chapter 22.) Hypomanic persons can avoid treatment for weeks, even months, consequently ruining their financial status, credit rating, employment history, relationships, and health.

As we shall see in a later section, many patients go through episodes of hypomania only and never become completely manic. Others have both hypomanic and manic episodes. Observations about the frequency and intensity of hypomanic versus manic episodes in different individuals are beginning to suggest that the classic "manic-depressive disorder" with episodes of full-blown mania and depression may be only one of many forms of the illness. (We shall discuss this new way of thinking about bipolar disorder in chapter 2, in the section "Bipolar Spectrum Disorders.")

The Syndrome of Depression

The depression of bipolar disorder is both easier and more difficult to describe and discuss than mania or hypomania. It is easier to discuss because depression is a more familiar set of feelings: everyone, whether suffering from bipolar disorder or not, has gone through periods of depressed mood. But the depressive syndrome of bipolar disorder is more difficult to discuss for that very reason: it is a very different experience from "normal" depression. In modern psychiatric terminology, this abnormal depressed mood state is called *major depression.*

When persons who do not suffer from a mood disorder go though a period of low mood, such as after a romantic disappointment, the loss of a job, or a period of homesickness, not only is their depressed mood temporary, but they retain the normal *reactivity* of mood. Anyone who has attended a funeral and then returned to the home of the bereaved afterward has probably observed this normal reactivity of mood, perhaps even in themselves. Mourners who might have been grief-stricken during the funeral service or at the grave site can afterward often relax, reminisce about good times with the person who has died, and enjoy catching up with friends and relatives perhaps not seen for a long time. The reactivity of mood is also retained in the lonely or homesick person who goes to the movies and loses himself or herself in a good film. We are able to dispel the feelings of bereavement, isolation, or disap-

TABLE 1-3 Symptoms of Depression

Mood Symptoms	*Bodily Symptoms*
Depressed mood	Sleep disturbance:
Dysphoric mood	insomnia
Diurnal variation of mood (early-morning depression, mood improving as day goes on)	hypersomnia
	Appetite disturbance:
	weight loss
	weight gain
Guilty feelings	Loss of interest in sex
Loss of ability to feel pleasure (anhedonia)	Fatigue
Social withdrawal	Constipation
Suicidal thoughts	Headaches
	Worsening of painful conditions
Cognitive (Thinking) Symptoms	
Poor concentration	*Symptoms of Psychosis*
Poor memory	Delusional thinking
Indecision	Hallucinations
Slowed thinking	Catatonic states

pointment—even if it's only for a few hours—if the depressed mood is a "normal" one.

The most significant feature of the depressed mood of the syndrome of depression is that instead of being reactive, the mood is *constricted*. Years ago AM radio stations used to give away free radios, gifts that came with only one catch: they couldn't be tuned to any of the sponsoring station's competitors. These radios were built to receive only the signal of the station that gave them away. The mood state of the person suffering through a depressed episode of bipolar disorder is like one of those radios, "set" to receive only one mood signal: depression. The mood of the syndrome of depression is a relentless, pervasive gloom that continues from one day to the next and from which the afflicted person cannot rouse himself or herself. As Pulitzer Prize–winning novelist William Styron said of his own depression, "The weather of depression is unmodulated, its light a brownout."[22]

In these constricted mood states, depressed individuals can find their thinking dominated by thoughts of sadness and loss, regret and hopelessness. Guilty ruminations are especially characteristic of the syndrome of depression, and psychiatrists often make a special point to ask about guilty feelings when examining a person being evaluated for depression. Ruminations on themes of guilt, shame, and regret are common in the depressed states of the mood disorders, and they are uncommon in "normal" depression. Persons experiencing the normal depressed mood that comes after a personal loss usually attribute their bad feelings to the fact that a loss has occurred; only in unusual circumstances will they feel that they are to blame for their problem and be preoccupied by guilty feelings or feelings of shame. The individual with a depressive syndrome, on the other hand, frequently feels to blame for his or her troubles, and sometimes for other peoples' troubles as well. The presence of guilty preoccupations is very significant for making a diagnosis of the syndrome of depression.

Feelings of inadequacy and worthlessness are similarly significant and especially common in the syndrome of major depression. Psychologist Norman Endler described how depression caused him to be tormented by feelings of incompetence even at the height of a successful academic career:

> [When I became depressed] I was positive I was a fraud and a phony
> and that I didn't deserve my Ph.D. I didn't deserve to have tenure;
> I didn't deserve to be a Full Professor; I didn't deserve to be a Fellow of
> the American Psychological Association and the Canadian Psycho-
> logical Association; I didn't deserve the research grants I had been
> awarded; I couldn't understand how I had written the books and jour-
> nal articles that I had and how they had been accepted for publication.
> I must have conned a lot of people.[23]

Another typical symptom of major depression is the loss of interest in usually pleasurable activities. This can be understood as another aspect of the loss of normal reactivity of mood. The depressed person is unable to derive any pleasure from listening to music, going to a movie, engaging in the sports or hobbies that usually provide enjoyment. This loss of the ability to feel pleasure has come to be called *anhedonia* (derived from the Greek word for "pleasure"). In his novel *The Sorrows of Young Werther*, Johann Wolfgang von Goethe has his main character express a loss of responsiveness to the joys and beauty of nature by saying, "Nature lies before me as immobile as in a little lacquered painting, and all this beauty cannot pump one drop of happiness from my heart to my brain."[24] Patients describe food losing its taste, colors draining away from sunrises and landscapes, flowers losing their textures and perfumes—everything becoming bland, dull, and lifeless. For some, the bright and beautiful things of the world become a source of anguish rather than pleasure. The nineteenth-century Austrian composer Hugo Wolf described a terrible sense of sorrowful isolation during his depressions, a feeling of separation from the world of ordinary pleasures—all the more painful when it occurred in springtime:

> What I suffer from . . . I am quite unable to describe. This wonderful spring with its secret life and movement troubles me unspeakably. These eternal blue skies, lasting for weeks, this continuous sprouting and budding in nature, these coaxing breezes impregnated with spring sunlight and fragrance of flowers . . . make me frantic. Everywhere this bewildering urge for life, fruitfulness, creation—and only I . . . may not take part in this festival of resurrection, at any rate not except as a spectator with grief and envy.[25]

Just as the manic syndrome infuses the affected person with feelings of inexpressible joy, the syndrome of depression brings indescribable anguish. Many individuals who have suffered from depression have struggled to describe the feelings, and even great writers seem to falter in the attempt. Quoting William Styron again: "If the pain were readily describable most of the countless sufferers from this ancient affliction would have been able to confidently depict . . . their torment. Healthy people [cannot] imagine a form of torment so alien to everyday experience. For myself, the pain is most closely connected to drowning or suffocation—but even these images are off the mark."[26]

Sometimes the "indescribable" mental discomfort seen in major depression is a feeling that seems different from the sad, pessimistic mood people usually mean by the word *depression*. Instead, people with major depression may have a tense, irritable, miserable sort of mood called *dysphoria*. (Remember that the term *dysphoric mania* is used to describe a tense, unpleasant, irritable mood that can be seen along with the agitation and hyperactivity of the manic state.)

The changes in thinking and physical well-being caused by the syndrome of depression are perhaps easier to describe. Energy level and thinking as well as mood are affected—in an opposite direction of polarity from that seen in mania. The depressed person experiences slowing and inefficiency in thinking and a feebleness of memory and concentration. Information processing and reasoning falter, and simple decisions can become overwhelming dilemmas. Quoting Endler again: "My indecisiveness was the worst of all. I couldn't decide what to eat or what to wear. I couldn't decide whether to get out of bed or to stay. I couldn't decide whether to shower or not to shower. I could never decide what to do because I didn't know myself."[27]

These *cognitive* functions (from the Latin *cognoscere,* meaning "to know") become progressively debilitated as the depression deepens, but even in milder depressions, ordinary mental tasks seem to require extraordinary effort. Kraepelin described the severe cognitive slowing he observed in his severely depressed patients: "[The patient's] thoughts are as if paralysed . . . immobile. He is no longer able to perceive or to follow the train of thought of a book or conversation . . . he has no memory, he has no longer command of knowledge formerly familiar to him [and] must consider a long time about simple things."[28] In the elderly, these sorts of thinking problems can be so severe that depression is misdiagnosed as Alzheimer's disease.

Severe depression almost always causes a change in sleeping pattern. Depressed persons frequently suffer from insomnia—but also from its opposite, sleeping too much (*hypersomnia* is the technical term). In the depression associated with bipolar disorder, hypersomnia seems especially common, perhaps more common than in other types of depression, where insomnia predominates.

There is sometimes seen in depressed persons a peculiar rhythmic pattern of sleep disturbance and mood changes throughout the day, called *diurnal variation of mood* (*diurnal* is a word used in biology to refer to a twenty-four-hour cycle). Persons with this pattern fall asleep at the usual time and without much difficulty but wake up very early in the morning after only a few hours of sleep. Lying awake hours before sunrise, they experience their lowest mood of the day, and minor problems and regrets seem magnified and overwhelming during this early-morning period. I recall one patient who told me that during those early-morning hours, "I lie awake thinking about every stupid thing I've ever done in my life." American author F. Scott Fitzgerald, who described his struggles with depression in the 1936 autobiographical work *The Crackup,* gave a vivid account of this mood pattern. He experienced the worst of his moods during the predawn hours, recalling that "at three o'clock in the morning, a forgotten package has the same tragic importance as a death sentence." For Fitzgerald, these nocturnal agonies were the worst part of his depressions, which he called "the dark night of the soul."[29] Individuals notice a gradual lifting of their mood as sunrise approaches, and when the morning light comes they can often rouse themselves and start their daily activities. As the day goes on, their mood continues to improve little by little until by day's end they feel nearly back to normal. They go to bed and can often fall asleep normally, but several hours later, it's "three o'clock in the morning" again: they awaken depressed, and the cycle repeats itself.

Novelist William Styron experienced a very striking diurnal variation in his mood during his depression, but with a reversal of the usual pattern: "While I was able to rise and function almost normally during the earlier part of the day, I began to sense the onset of the symptoms at mid-afternoon or a little later—gloom crowding in on me, a sense of dread and alienation and . . . stifling anxiety."[30]

The disruptions of various bodily rhythms that occur in depression and mania have convinced many scientists that some persons with mood disorders have a disturbance of their *chronobiology* (from *chronos,* the Greek word for "time"). Persons with mood disorders have been observed to have disturbances in the normal rhythmic pulsing of various hormone levels, in body temperature fluctuations, the sleep-wake cycle, and other natural rhythms. Later in this book we shall examine connections between these natural rhythms and mood and shall look at other cycles: the monthly cycles of mood in women with premenstrual mood symptoms (chapter 14) and the twelve-month cycles of persons with seasonal affective disorder (chapter 16).

Appetite is usually disturbed in depressed individuals. As with sleep problems, changes occur in both directions, and patients may eat too much or too little. Individuals can lose or gain a significant amount of weight during periods of depression. As might be expected, the depressed person loses interest in sex, perhaps best understood as part of his or her inability to experience pleasurable activities of any kind, the "anhedonia" of depression.

Of the other bodily symptoms that occur in depression, a sense of fatigue with prominent low energy and listlessness is one of the most striking. Here is Endler: "[My] fatigue [was] extreme to the point of exhaustion. I was too tired to make decisions and felt as if I had a huge weight on my back that wouldn't allow me to achieve anything . . . No matter how long I stayed in bed and slept I never felt rested and refreshed . . . When I did get out of bed I was lethargic. I was slow as molasses."[31] Headaches, constipation, and a feeling of heaviness in the chest are common, as are other more difficult-to-describe sensations of physical discomfort. Here is Styron: "I felt a kind of numbness, an enervation . . . an odd fragility—as if my body had actually become frail, hypersensitive and somehow disjointed and clumsy. Nothing felt quite right

. . . there were twitches and pains, sometimes intermittent, often seemingly constant, that seemed to presage all sorts of dire infirmities."[32]

It is not clear whether these symptoms are caused by depression itself or arise from the lack of restful sleep, the lack of exercise, and the poor eating habits that depression brings on. Persons who have preexisting painful medical conditions such as arthritis or inflammatory bowel disease are usually more bothered by the physical symptoms of these illnesses when they are depressed. The connections between depression and problems with fatigue seen in chronic fatigue immunodeficiency syndrome (CFIDS) and the painful joint and muscle disease fibromyalgia are well known but poorly understood. Depression seems to lower the pain threshold: depressed individuals seem more sensitive to pain and are more distressed by it.

Some persons may be willing to seek treatment for these physical symptoms but reluctant to mention their mood problems. This can cause patients with depression to end up getting all kinds of tests and treatments for physical illnesses from their physicians when their real problem is depression.

Just as in the syndrome of mania, persons suffering through an episode of the depression of bipolar disorder can experience the distortions of thinking that psychiatrists call *delusions*. As their view of the world and of themselves is increasingly colored by their pervasive mood changes, depressed individuals can come to believe that terrible things are happening all around them: "I was positive that I was going to be fired from the university because of incompetence and that [my family] would become destitute—that we would go broke," wrote Endler. "I felt guilty at the prospect of not being able to support my family."[33] In addition to such *delusions of poverty,* delusions can arise from the uncomfortable physical sensations of depression. Patients believe they have cancer, AIDS, or some other terrible illness. Kraepelin described the increasingly bizarre *hypochondriacal delusions* he sometimes observed in his patients: "[The patient believes he is] incurably ill, half-dead, no longer a right human being, has lung disease, a tapeworm, cancer in his throat, cannot swallow, does not retain his food . . . Face and figure have changed; there is no longer blood in his brain, he does not see any longer, must become crazy, remain his whole lifetime in an institution, die, has already died." Patients with these sorts of beliefs may refuse to eat or drink, convinced that their body cannot absorb the food. *Paranoid delusions,* beliefs that one is in danger or the victim of evil people and forces, can also occur. Quoting Kraepelin again:

Everywhere danger threatens the patient . . . strange people are in the house; a suspicious motorcar drives past. People mock him, are going to thrash him, to chase him from his post in a shameful way, incarcerate him, bring him to justice, expose him publicly, deport him, throw him into the fire, drown him. The people are already standing outside; the bill of indictment is already written; the scaffold is being put up; he must wander about naked and miserable . . . His relatives also are being tortured . . . his family is imprisoned, his wife has drowned herself; his parents are murdered; his daughter wanders about in the snow without any clothes on.[34]

It's easy to understand why suicidal thinking and behavior are so common in the syndrome of major depression: compared with the horrors of such delusional imaginings, death may seem a welcome alternative. It's also possible to understand why delusionally depressed persons can occasionally be dangerous to others as well as to themselves: delusionally depressed individuals can come to believe that those close to them are in similar danger of gruesome persecution and would be better off dead.

Hallucinations occur in severe depressions, but not as frequently as in mania. The hallucinations are consistent with the mood and are frightening, even horrifying: "The patients see evil spirits, death, heads of animals . . . crowds of monsters . . . dead relatives . . . The patient hears his tortured relatives screaming and lamenting . . . his food tastes of soapy water or excrement, of corpses and mildew."[35]

Some seriously ill patients sink into a state of lethargy and despair that is called *depressive stupor.* Styron's description of this horrible condition is the best I have ever read:

I had now reached that phase of the disorder where all sense of hope had vanished, along with the idea of a futurity; my brain . . . had become less an organ of thought than an instrument registering,

TABLE 1-4 Delusions and Hallucinations in Bipolar Disorder: Mania versus Depression

Category of Symptoms	Percentage of Patients
Delusions	
Mania	44
Depression	12
Hallucinations	
Mania	14
Depression	8

Source: Data from D. W. Black and A. Nasrallah, "Hallucinations and Delusions in 1,715 Patients with Unipolar and Bipolar Affective Disorders," *Psychopathology* 22 (1989): 28–34.

minute by minute, varying degrees of its own suffering . . . I'd feel the horror, like some poisonous fog bank, roll in upon my mind, forcing me to bed. There I would lie for as long as six hours, stuporous and virtually paralyzed, gazing at the ceiling.[36]

Just as few modern psychiatrists have ever seen the most extreme stage of mania, so-called *delirious mania*, it is also fortunately rare today to see a patient depressed to the point of unresponsiveness and immobility that psychiatrists call *catatonia*. Kraepelin, describing patients of an era when virtually no treatment was available for this terrible condition, starkly describes the deepest abyss of depression: "The patients lie in bed taking no interest in anything. They betray no pronounced emotion; they are mute, inaccessible; they pass their [bowel movements] under them; they stare straight in front of them with [a] vacant expression of countenance like a mask and with wide open eyes."[37]

Electroconvulsive therapy (ECT), which we shall discuss in more detail in chapter 10, is a very effective treatment for these extreme states of the depressive syndrome. Although there have been misguided attempts to ban this safe and effective treatment technique in the United States, and equally misguided activists still occasionally appear in the media to disparage ECT, it fortunately remains available to treat this most extreme stage of depression, rescuing these individuals from a kind of living hell.

Mixed Mood States

There is another type of abnormal mood occasionally seen in bipolar disorder, a strange combination of both the frenzied intensity of mania and the horrors of deep depression that has been called a *mixed state* (sometimes, *mixed affective state*). Kay Jamison described these states as the most terrible expression of the illness for her: "On occasion, these periods of total despair would be made even worse by terrible agitation. My mind would race from subject to subject, but instead of being filled with . . . exuberance and cosmic thoughts . . . it would be drenched in awful sounds and images of decay and dying; dead bodies on the beach, charred remains of animals, toe-tagged corpses in morgues."[38]

Although psychiatrists do not yet agree on the defining characteristics for this mood state, they have long recognized that symptoms of depression and mania seem to exist almost simultaneously in some patients. A seventeenth-century English physician observed rapidly alternating symptoms of mania and depression, noting that "they succeed each other in a double and alternate act; or take each other's place like the smoke and flame of fire."[39] Kraepelin described six types of mixed states, giving them labels such as "anxious mania" and "excited depression."[40]

TABLE 1-5 Symptoms in Ten Patients with Mixed Mania (Dysphoric Mania)

Symptoms	Percentage of Patients
Depressed mood	100
Irritable mood	100
Increased activity	100
Insomnia	93
Pressured speech	93
Hostility	79
Flight of ideas	43
Anxiety attacks	43
Delusions (depressive)	36
Delusions (nondepressive)	21

Source: Data from Frederick K. Goodwin and Kay Redfield Jamison, *Manic-Depressive Illness* (New York: Oxford University Press, 1990), 49.

Because some patients in an otherwise typical manic episode develop desperate, anxious, distraught symptoms as they become sicker, one can make a case for the "mixed" state being called a stage of mania ("stage III mania" as described earlier in this chapter in the section on mania). But there seem to be other patients for whom this mixed state represents a distinct variety of abnormal mood separate from both depression and typical mania. In these patients the accelerated thinking and hyperactivity typical of the manic state remain a striking feature, but they are combined with a depressed, despairing, desperate mood. Kraepelin described patients with "flight of ideas, excitement and anxiety" who were "anxiously despairing."[41] The labels now being used most frequently for the mixed state are "mixed mania" and "dysphoric mania."[42] As we shall see in chapter 2, there is some evidence that this mood state does not occur in all patients with bipolar disorder, and that when it does occur, a different treatment approach is necessary.

Another type of mood "mixture" occurs when, rather than a true mixture of mania and depression simultaneously, there is very rapid alternation between the two states. Kraepelin described "transition periods from one state to another, which often [extended] over weeks" during which his patients seemed depressed one moment and manic nearly the next:

Manic patients may transitorily appear not only sad and despairing, but also quiet and inhibited. A patient goes to bed moody and inhibited, suddenly wakes up with the feeling as if a veil had been drawn away from his brain, passes the day in manic delight in work, and the next morning, exhausted and with a heavy head, he again finds in himself the whole misery of his state. Or the hypomanic exultant patient quite unexpectedly makes a serious attempt at suicide.[43]

Recently the term *ultra-rapid cycling* has been proposed for these rapid alternations in mood seen in some bipolar patients.

Now that you have some familiarity with the symptoms of bipolar disorder, I can talk about diagnosis. As I have already said, most people with bipolar disorder never develop all the possible symptoms of the illness. It is the presence or absence of certain symptoms as well as the *pattern* of mood symptoms that allows a diagnosis of a particular type of bipolar disorder to be made. And once a diagnosis has been made, a treatment plan can be developed. In the next chapter you'll see how the diagnostic process works.

Although the same morbid process lies at the foundation of all these forms [of manic-depressive illness], they are yet so different in clinical behavior, in course, and in prognosis, that one might perhaps speak of a morbid group springing from a common root.

EMIL KRAEPELIN

The Diagnosis of Bipolar Disorder

WHEN LITHIUM BECAME AVAILABLE IN THE 1970S AS A TREATMENT FOR bipolar disorder, psychiatrists started to realize that not all cases of bipolar disorder were the same. For some patients, lithium was indeed a miracle; their symptoms were completely controlled by it, and their illness seemed simply to end. But other patients—often those with more severe symptoms and more frequent episodes of abnormal mood—didn't respond as well to the medication. Did these people have bipolar disorder, or something else? Patients who had been thought to have "cyclothymic personality disorder"—a diagnostic category in an old edition of the diagnostic manual of the American Psychiatric Association—also saw their troublesome and unpredictable mood variations stop when they took lithium; did these people have bipolar disorder, and not a personality problem after all? Was this a milder form of "manic-depressive" illness, or a different disorder altogether? Did it matter? What difference does diagnosis make, anyway?

Diagnostic classification has two purposes in medicine: to make predictions about the course of an illness, and to aid the clinician in selecting the treatment most likely to be effective. In the practice of psychiatry, since the physical basis for most psychiatric illnesses has yet to be discovered, classification systems are largely derived from studying groups of patients with different combinations of symptoms and seeing if the different groups vary in the course of their illness or in their response to medications.

As lithium and other medications have become available to treat mood disorders, the classification system for bipolar mood disorders has continued to evolve. In the sections that follow, various subtypes of bipolar disorder are described. These are the subtypes that currently seem to make sense to clinicians because they serve one of the two purposes of diagnosis mentioned above: they allow for a better prediction of the course of the illness, and they allow for a rapid selection of effective therapy—saving the patient time that would be wasted on a trial of an ineffective medication.

Psychiatric Diagnosis

At least once a month, it seems, I see a patient who asks to be "tested for bipolar disorder." It's not an unreasonable request. Unfortunately, it's not a request that can be satisfied—not just yet. There's not a blood test or an x-ray or a biopsy that can make the diagnosis of bipolar disorder (or, for that matter, that can be used to confirm the diagnosis of most of the problems psychiatrists treat).

The reason for this sorry state of affairs is that the biological and chemical basis of bipolar disorder remains a nearly complete mystery; no one knows what to test for. Despite literally hundreds of years of examining the bodily fluids and brain tissues of individuals with mood disorders—first with the naked eye, then with microscopes, later with x-rays and scanning devices, and more recently with incredibly sophisticated biochemical probes—no one has been able to find in patients with this illness any abnormalities that can be accurately and reliably measured as an aid in diagnosing the disorder. Although work in the genetics of bipolar disorder holds the promise that genetic markers for the illness may be discovered in the not too distant future—suggesting that a blood test might be possible that will identify at least some cases of the illness—and although some individuals with bipolar disorder have been identified as having subtle brain-scan abnormalities (see "Picturing Bipolar Disorder in the Brain" in chapter 18), again suggesting a possible diagnostic tool, the clinical applications of these findings are still far off. Modern psychiatrists are left with the same diagnostic tools that Emil Kraepelin and other nineteenth-century psychiatrists had: their eyes and ears.

We psychiatrists listen to the patient and to his or her family members describe symptoms—their onset, course, fluctuation, and impact upon the patient. We observe the patient for the signs of bipolar disorder described in chapter 1 by performing a *mental status examination,* the psychiatrist's equivalent of the physical examination; this examination consists of observing speech patterns and behavior, asking questions about mood and thinking processes, and evaluating other aspects of mental functioning such as concentration and memory. After this process of history taking and examination, a picture of the person and of his or her symptoms and the course of the trouble emerges. A particular diagnostic category that seems to be a good fit with the clinical information is identified. Once the diagnostic category of the illness is determined, we can make predictions about the future course of the symptoms and, perhaps more important, can select a treatment that has a good chance of relieving them. In the sections that follow we shall learn about the different forms of bipolar disorder the same way young physicians training to be psychiatrists do: by hearing from patients.

Bipolar I

It had been several years since I had seen Richard in the mood-disorders clinic. He looked great. Although he was only in his late thirties, some silver tones in his hair made him look a bit older and quite distinguished. I remembered that he had always dressed well, but today, in an obviously finely tailored suit, a crisp white shirt, and beautiful silk tie, he looked—well, like a million. I knew that this could be a very good sign—or a very bad sign.

"That's a handsome suit you've got on, Richard. Is it new?" I asked.

"I got it about a month ago," he said proudly, "in London. A terrific shop on Savile Row, the same one Prince Charles goes to." He smiled a little mischievously. "And I know what you're thinking: no, I wasn't manic when I bought it!"

Rich certainly knew what mania was, as did several members of his family. His wealthy parents had taken control of his financial affairs in a legal-guardianship proceeding; for years he hadn't even been able to write a check at the supermarket. Rich had first developed manic symptoms during law school, making down payments on not just one Porsche but three before a check bounced. He had angrily stormed into the bank's branch office to protest, created quite a scene, and ended up in jail, where an astute nurse fortunately arranged an immediate psychiatric evaluation. Richard was in a local psychiatric hospital and had taken his first dose of lithium before his parents even knew what had happened.

He stopped taking his lithium within a month of leaving the hospital and started having manic symptoms almost immediately. This time his manic enthusiasm turned to travel rather than cars, and he used a credit card to buy an airline ticket to Fiji. He made it as far as Los Angeles before his mania turned dysphoric and irritable again. He had started yelling at and shoving a security guard who wanted to examine his luggage and wound up in jail again—this time with federal charges. After a talk with a good lawyer, another hospitalization, more lithium, a leave from law school, and a move back home, he had come for treatment at the university outpatient clinic where I was training.

Richard's father also suffered from bipolar disorder and knew, from his own turbulent experiences with the illness, just how to handle the situation. A pair of scissors to the credit cards, a power of attorney, and going along with Richard to the psychiatrist's appointments made the difference—as did the fact that Richard was an intelligent fellow who (eventually) learned from experience as well. Moreover, he learned from his father that a paternal uncle who had been killed in a car accident when Rich was a child had also actually probably died from the disease; the single-passenger accident had most likely been a suicide. Rich made the decision to take control of the illness rather than let it control him. And as with most things, once he decided to do so, Rich applied himself to staying well with energy and determination.

There was a time after he broke up with a girlfriend when severe depressive symptoms almost necessitated another hospitalization for Rich; he spent fourteen to sixteen hours in bed every day for nearly three weeks and put on almost fifty pounds. Fortunately, family support, an excellent psychologist in the clinic who saw him for therapy, and a higher lithium dose for several months got him through. After about a year of stable mood, he got into a local law school to finish his studies and eventually graduated at the top of his class. He had taken a job in New York but now had returned home. "I couldn't pass up the opportunity to open my firm's new branch office in my hometown, could I?" he beamed.

Rich brought me up to date. A little hypomania had occasionally emerged during the summers while he was working in New York, especially if he was working too hard and didn't watch his sleep habits. But Rich had obviously remained serious about his mental health; he monitored his moods and saw his psychiatrist regularly. Most important, he was making career decisions that reflected his knowledge of his illness. "I think the pace will be slower here than in New York. I may not become a millionaire as quickly," he said a little sadly, "but there will also be less risk of getting sick, blowing it all, and having to start over again. So . . . I had my last lithium level done three months ago, and it was 0.8. When do you want me to get another?"

It looked as if the suit had been a very *good* sign.

Bipolar I is the designation for the classic variety of bipolar disorder, characterized by full-blown manic attacks and deep, paralysing depressions. A schematic representation of the moods of bipolar I appears in figure 2-1. The

FIGURE 2-1 Mood changes in bipolar I

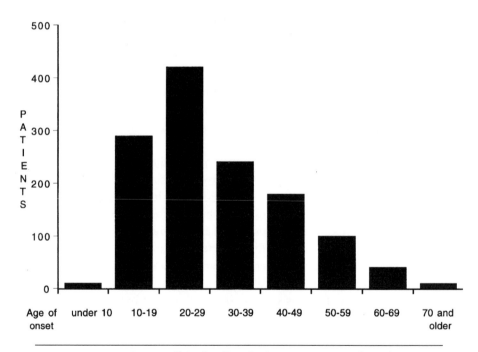

FIGURE 2-2 Age of onset of bipolar disorder in 1,304 patients. These data were compiled from ten different studies carried out between 1969 and 1984. Notice that early adulthood is the peak time for the onset of the disorder.

Source: Frederick K. Goodwin and Kay Redfield Jamison, *Manic-Depressive Illness* (New York: Oxford University Press, 1990), 132. Copyright © 1990 by Oxford University Press, Inc. Used by permission of Oxford University Press, Inc.

pattern of abnormal mood episodes seems to vary widely, and the rhythm of the illness is almost as individual as the patient who has it. Symptoms of bipolar I usually begin in the late teens or early twenties, although onset at later ages is not uncommon.[1]

Bipolar I is what physicians refer to as a relapsing and remitting illness; during the course of the illness, its symptoms come and go. This feature of bipolar I—it is actually a feature of *all* mood disorders—makes it difficult to diagnose, difficult to treat, and fiendishly difficult to study. This deserves a closer look.

THE DISEASE THAT SLEEPS

When we think about illnesses of the body, we usually think of diseases that have a beginning, a middle, and an end. Take, for example, pneumonia, an infection of the lungs caused by bacteria. The disease begins when fever, cough, chest pains, and breathing problems appear. These symptoms build and worsen over a period of hours or sometimes days. Before the antibiotic era, patients reached what was called a *crisis* point, when their bodies' natural defenses had mounted their best effort against the bacterial invaders, and the patient either started getting better or died. Either the patient killed off the bacteria or vice-versa, but in any case the disease process came to an end. (Fortunately we can now administer antibiotics that usually give the patient's defenses the crucial edge against the bacterial invader.)

How about a disease not caused by a foreign invader like bacteria but instead one in which the body seems to turn on itself, a disease like cancer—say, leukemia? In this case a white blood cell in the body develops an abnormality that causes it to start reproducing uncontrollably. Most of the cells in the body reproduce from time to time, in order to replenish those that wear out. It is thought that most cancers are caused by an error during cell duplication that results in an abnormality in the control center of one of the new cells, probably involving DNA. This abnormality causes the cell to start reproducing continuously. More and more abnormal cells are produced, and in the case of leukemia they fill the bloodstream and lymph nodes such that the normal cells cannot do their job properly, the immune system fails, and the patient dies. Many types of leukemia are now curable. The cures basically involve using ingenious methods to eradicate every single cancer cell, eliminating the abnormally reproducing cells altogether; when the abnormality is eliminated from the body, things return to normal. Again, the illness begins when something goes wrong in the body, and it ends (is cured) when the abnormality is corrected and eliminated. The illness is finished for good.

Bipolar disorder is very different from these diseases because it does not simply have a beginning, a middle, and an end. Or perhaps it is more accurate to say that the illness seems to have many beginnings and endings: the symptoms of bipolar disorder can develop in an individual, and then *without any treatment at all* the symptoms may go away for years at a time—a pattern that is nearly unique among the diseases that afflict humankind.

Since most people are more familiar with diseases that end when their symptoms go away, it is often very difficult for patients and their families to understand that although the symptoms of bipolar disorder can go into *remission* after treatment (or even spontaneously), they almost inevitably will come back if treatment to prevent their return is not in place. The hallmark of bipolar illness—especially bipolar I—is the tendency of the illness to *relapse.* No matter how well the symptoms of any one episode are treated, the illness does not end but instead seems merely to hibernate—and *symptoms can come back at any time.*

THE NATURAL HISTORY OF BIPOLAR I

Now, back to a description of the characteristics of bipolar I. Fortunately many excellent clinical studies about the course of bipolar disorder were done in the years before effective treatments for it were available; these studies document and illustrate the pattern of bipolar-disorder symptoms that exists if the illness is not treated—what physicians call the *natural history* of the illness.[2]

How many episodes of illness did patients have in the days before treatment was available? How long did episodes last? What was the length of time between episodes?

In a 1942 study, the records of sixty-six patients with "manic-depressive psychosis" were studied; some of these individuals had been followed for up to twenty-six years. Although a few patients seemed to have had only one episode of illness in the period of study, about one-third had two to three episodes, about one-third had four to six episodes, and about one-third had

TABLE 2-1 Number of Episodes of Illness in Sixty-six Patients with Bipolar Disorder

Number of Episodes	Percentage of Patients
1	8
2–3	29
4–6	26
More than 7	37

Source: Data from Thomas A. C. Rennie, "Prognosis in Manic-Depressive Psychosis," *American Journal of Psychiatry,* 98 (1942): 801–14.

Note: This study was done before the availability of any treatments for bipolar disorder.

more than seven. A few had twenty or more episodes.[3] Unfortunately, when a diagnosis of bipolar I is made, there is no way to know whether the individual will have another two or three episodes during his or her lifetime or more than twenty.

How long did episodes of mania or major depression last before effective treatments were available? In the 1942 study, the average duration was about six and a half months. But we also know that depressions and manias were sometimes shorter and sometimes lasted much longer. Kraepelin, writing at a time when there were essentially no effective treatments, noted that

> the duration of individual attacks is extremely varied. There are some which last only eight to fourteen days, indeed we sometimes see that states of moodiness or excitement . . . do not continue in these patients longer than one or two days or even only a few hours. For the most part, however, a simple attack usually lasts six to eight months. On the other hand, the cases are not at all rare, in which an attack continues for two, three or four years, and a double attack [can] double that time. I have seen manias, which even after seven years, indeed after more than ten years, recovered, and a state of depression which after fourteen years recovered.[4]

Modern psychiatrists no longer see patients who are manic for years at a time. Effective modern treatments abort these episodes, and the patient is usually better in a few days—weeks at the most. Modern psychiatrists do, however, see patients who seem to become manic again and again, month after month, year after year—often every time they stop taking medication. Do these patients have many episodes, or do they have many relapses of a single episode of several years' duration? I tend to think it's the latter, but the rhythm of the illness makes research very difficult.

How about the time between attacks? For many persons with bipolar disorder, modern treatments are quite effective at keeping the episodes from recurring. But how long did remissions last in the days before these treatments were available? Kraepelin noted that the time between episodes could be years, even decades. Among 703 "intervals" that he studied in his patients, Kraepelin found one case in which forty-four years separated one episode of illness from the next.[5] However, many subsequent studies have shown that, if untreated, episodes of bipolar disorder occur more and more frequently in individual patients. The illness seems to accelerate if untreated, and in the days before treatment was available, mood episodes tended to recur more and more frequently as patients aged. This acceleration has profound implications for treatment and prognosis, as we shall see in chapter 20.

Another finding in these older studies is that some patients tend to "switch" from a depression to a manic episode without an interval of normal

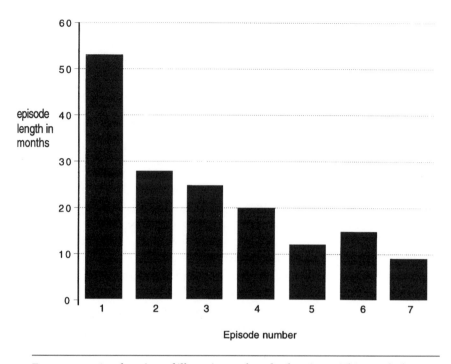

FIGURE 2-3 Acceleration of illness in one hundred patients. This graph shows that the cycle length of episodes of bipolar disorder (the time from the onset of one episode to the onset of the next) becomes shorter and shorter in patients whose symptoms are not well controlled and who continue to have episodes of the illness.

Source: Data from P. P. Roy-Burne, R. M. Post, T. W. Uhde, T. Porcu, and D. Davis, "The Longitudinal Course of Recurrent Affective Illness: Life Chart Data from Patients at the NIMH," *Acta Psychiatrica Scandinavia* 71, suppl. 317 (1985): 1–34.

TABLE 2-2 Features of Bipolar I

Mood
Fully developed manic episodes
Fully developed depressive episodes

Other Features
Untreated episodes average six months
Hallucinations and delusions frequently seen
Triphasic episodes
Relapses more frequent as patient ages

mood. In a 1969 study, the course of one hundred manic episodes was described.[6] Many individuals were noted to have a period of depression of several weeks' or months' duration that switched into a manic episode, again of several months' duration. In a few of these patients, there followed another switch and the beginning of a third phase of the episode: a long period of depression. In this study, about half of the patients' manic episodes showed at least one switch—a depression either before or after their manic episode. There have been several studies that suggest that patients who "switch" from depression to mania have a more difficult-to-treat form of illness than those who switch from mania to depression.[7]

Bipolar I is the classic manic-depressive illness, with fully developed manic episodes and episodes of severe depression, and it is also characterized by long periods of "hibernation" in which the symptoms temporarily disappear. The number of episodes varies enormously, but patients who have only one or two episodes seem to be the exception rather than the rule. Before effective treatments became available, the average length of each episode if untreated was about six months—but episodes that lasted years were not at all uncommon.

Bipolar II

Robert was a thirty-nine-year-old accountant who had been seeing a psychologist for treatment of depression for about three months. Both he and his therapist were frustrated because despite the best efforts of both, Robert's depression seemed to be getting worse.

"I can usually pull myself out of these things—or at least I can usually slog through them until they finish," he told me at our first appointment. Right away, his description of his depressions as "these things" made me feel pretty certain that this fellow had a mood disorder. Robert's moods had an alien, external quality to him; they came upon him like a fog bank rolling in, lasted for a few weeks, and then slowly dissipated. Where they came from and where they went was a complete mystery to Robert. He would sleep away the weekends, put on weight, fall behind in his work. "This has been happening to me since college," he said, "and I really want it to stop." In fact, this was not the worst his depressions had ever gotten. Shortly after graduation, Robert had had such a severe depression that he had spent most of the summer at home in his room. At one point he had seriously contemplated suicide. The only reason he hadn't gotten into treatment then was because he had felt he was no worse off than his mother.

Robert's mother was a closet alcoholic. "There was always one of those huge bottles of wine in the refrigerator," he told me. "It always seemed either full or half full, and when I was in high school I realized that this was because she drank about a half a gallon every day." Robert's mother had never had any treatment for either her drinking problem or for depression, but his description of the long "naps" she took most afternoons and the "sick headaches" that put her in bed for weeks sounded like more than alcoholism—more like a smoldering depression *complicated* by alcohol addiction. Another red flag for a mood-disorder diagnosis: a positive family history.

Robert had always blamed his melancholic moods on his childhood. The memories of his shame and worry about his mother seeped back into his consciousness during these times, as did guilty feelings that he had put hundreds of miles between himself and his mother now, hadn't seen her in over two years, and could bring himself to call her only on holidays. Here was more evidence pointing to a mood disorder: guilty feelings and painful preoccupations with the past that seemed really to bother him only when his mood changed. Though I wasn't quite through taking his history, I was already thinking about which antidepressant to recommend to him when Robert gave me another piece of information that changed everything.

"I even feel like my *thinking* is slower than usual. I'll never get through tax season unless I do something to get some help—or unless one of my highs kicks in."

"One of your . . . ?"

"I call it a high. But it's not like I'm manic-depressive or anything. It's just that sometimes when things get back to normal I'm so relieved and happy that—oh, I don't know, it just feels so good not to be depressed."

"Do you find that you're especially productive during these times?" I asked.

"Oh, definitely. One year I came out of a depression just in time for tax season. I didn't feel overwhelmed like I usually do. It was spring, and I wasn't depressed for a change, and I had just met the girl I was going to marry—in fact we got married that summer, and so of course things settled back down. But that was a great year."

"Do other people notice?"

"Um, yes, especially at the office. 'Slow down, Rob.' 'Take it easy, Rob.' Sometimes I get irritated by that."

I had a few more questions to ask, but I was beginning to think about how to tell this fellow that he probably had "manic-depression" after all.

Time ⟶

FIGURE 2-4 Mood changes in bipolar II

Bipolar II is characterized by fully developed depressive episodes and episodes of *hypo*mania. A schematic representation of the moods of bipolar II appears in figure 2-4.

When lithium became available in the United States in the 1970s and researchers were trying to find better diagnostic criteria for bipolar disorder, several of them noticed that there was a large group of patients who didn't have a history of fully developed manic episodes but who seemed to be bipolar nonetheless. They had severe depressions, but their "highs" never developed into mania. Were these patients "manic-depressives" who were still early in the course of their illness and simply hadn't had time to have a fully developed manic episode? Several studies attempting to answer this question concluded that these patients did *not* usually go on to fully developed mania. In one study, fewer than 5 percent of the patients with recurrent depressions and hypomania ever became manic.[8] Several studies showed as well that these patients often had relatives who also had a bipolar mood disorder characterized by major depressions and hypomanias.[9] Although patients with bipolar II sometimes have family members who have bipolar I or depressive disorders (without either mania or hypomania), the disorder frequently seems to "breed true": family members of persons with bipolar II who have mood disorders also tend to have bipolar II symptom patterns.[10]

Since bipolar II is a rather new way of classifying bipolar disorders, we can't go back into the research literature of the days before lithium and look for statistics on the course of untreated bipolar II. So we don't know for sure if bipolar II patients have longer or shorter or more frequent or less frequent episodes of illness. Nevertheless, modern studies indicate that there are a few typical features of bipolar II.

Bipolar II patients seem to have more problems with depression—in fact the depression is sometimes so prominent that many receive a diagnosis of depressive disorder and don't get treatment for bipolar disorder at all. In a study from the National Institutes of Health published in 1995, 559 patients diagnosed with a depressive disorder were followed over time, some for up to eleven years. It was reported that almost 9 percent of them developed symptoms of bipolar II.[11] The first hypomanic episode could usually be documented within several months of the onset of severe depression, but sometimes it took up to nine years for the correct diagnosis to become clear. Some of these 559 "depression" patients also developed a manic episode—that is, they turned out to have bipolar I—but this was far less common (only 3.9 percent). This study also found that bipolar II patients had longer depressive episodes (52.2 weeks) than bipolar I patients (24.3 weeks). Bipolar II patients have also been found to be at higher risk for alcoholism.[12]

What is the relationship between bipolar I and bipolar II? At present, there are only interesting speculations. As noted above, it is fairly clear that bipolar II is not merely a prelude to "full-blown" manic-depressive illness—that is, bipolar II patients are not in the early stages of bipolar I. These two conditions really seem to be separate illnesses, and bipolar II can perhaps best be thought of as a milder form of bipolar I.

There is some evidence to suggest that bipolar II is actually more common than bipolar I. Researchers from Johns Hopkins University published a study in 1993 showing that when the family members of individuals with bipolar disorder (I or II) are evaluated for mood disorders, bipolar II shows up most often.[13] Even when family members of individuals with bipolar I were studied, bipolar II was more frequent.

These researchers suggested that instead of thinking of bipolar II as a less

TABLE 2-3 Features of Bipolar II

Mood

Fully developed depressive episodes
Hypomanic episodes

Other Features

Increased sleep and appetite during depressions
Depressions sometimes more chronic
Bipolar II history in family members
Later age at first hospitalization
Fewer hospitalizations
Possible increased risk for alcoholism

TABLE 2-4 Family Histories of Bipolar I and Bipolar II Patients

	Family Members of Bipolar I Patients	Family Members of Bipolar II Patients
Percentage diagnosed with bipolar I	15.5	2.1
Percentage diagnosed with bipolar II	22.4	40.4

Source: Data from Sylvia Simpson, Susan Folstein, Deborah Meyers, Francis McMahon, Diane Brusco, and J. Raymond DePaulo, "Bipolar II: The Most Common Bipolar Phenotype?" *American Journal of Psychiatry* 150 (1993): 901–3.

severe form of bipolar I, it might be more accurate to think of the relationship the other way round. Bipolar II might be the more common and "simpler" disorder, and bipolar I its more complicated and more severe form. Perhaps individuals with bipolar II, the simpler disorder, have only one mood-disorder gene. Bipolar I might be the result of multiple "hits," either when multiple genes are affected or because of some other combination of abnormal genes and environmental events.

Cyclothymic Disorder

Phil was a thirty-one-year-old recently married man whose wife had insisted that he come to the local community mental-health clinic because of his "mood swings." He had never had any psychiatric treatment before and wasn't sure he really needed any now. "I'm doing this for her, Doc. I'm not crazy," he said as he sat down. "If you really want to know, I think *she's* the one with the problem."

"What do you mean?"

"Well, don't get me wrong. She's a great girl, and I really love her, but . . ." He seemed to be having a hard time admitting something. "She's an only child, and she's—well, I admit it, she's more mature than I am, and she can't, oh, I don't know . . . just go with the flow."

I smiled a little and shook my head. "Sorry, Phil, I'm not getting it."

"Well, I don't think my mood swings are *that* bad. I think she's overreacting to them. Everyone has good days and bad, don't they?"

"Well, yes, that's true, of course, but some people seem to have runs of extremely good days and of extremely bad days that they can't quite account for. Have you ever experienced anything like that?"

In fact Phil never knew when he went to bed at night just what his mood might be when he got up. He sold expensive sailboats for a living and was usually good at it—in fact sometimes he was great at it, but he needed those "great" times to offset the down times. During the down times, which lasted up to a week, Phil would miss work, sleep ten to twelve hours a day, lose interest in everything—including sex with his wife—and be just miserable. Then he would suddenly awake one morning with boundless energy, confidence, and enthusiasm and sell more boats in two days than he had the previous week. But there was a down side to the "up" times too—sometimes Phil would get impatient with customers, pressure them too much, and lose a sale he might otherwise have made. He also drank too much during these times and had even been arrested once for "driving under the influence."

School had been similar: uneven and unpredictable performance. Sometimes he got A's and B's and other times D's and F's. His high school teachers thought him bright but "not mature enough for college" and suggested that he work for a few years before attempting it, perhaps thinking a dose of life in the "real world" would teach Phil better self-control.

"But I *can't* control how I feel; that's just the way I am. I've just learned how to live with it."

And this was, of course, exactly the point. Phil thought that everyone lived at the mercy of their moods and learned how to "go with the flow," as he put it—learned how to adjust his or her schedule and activities according to unpredictable fluctuations of mood. It was only when he got married that he got an objective observer—his wife—who noticed that Phil's moods had a life and rhythm of their own. "She keeps telling me that everyone *doesn't* have mood swings like I do, but I think she's wrong. What do you think?"

"Well, I think you married a very astute young woman. I think she might be right."

———————————————————————————————————

Cyclothymic disorder (-*thymia,* from the Greek word for "mind," is used in psychiatry to refer to mood) is characterized by frequent short periods (days to weeks) of depressive symptoms and of hypomania separated by periods (which also tend to be short, on the order of days to weeks) of fairly normal mood. By definition, the patient does not have either fully developed major depressive episodes or manic episodes. A schematic representation of the moods of cyclothymia appears in figure 2-5.

Emil Kraepelin believed that "there are certain temperaments which may be regarded as rudiments of manic-depressive insanity. They may [exist]

FIGURE 2-5 Mood changes in cyclothymia

throughout the whole of life as peculiar forms of psychic personality without further development." Kraepelin described "cyclothymic temperament" as "characterized by frequent, more or less regular fluctuations of the psychic state to the manic or to the depressive side."[14] He reported that 3 to 4 percent of his patients had the cyclothymic temperament but speculated that many more persons might have similar illnesses that "run their course outside of institutions." Modern research on community populations have proven Kraepelin (as usual) quite correct. Several studies have shown that cyclothymic disorder probably affects 3 to 6 percent of the population.[15] Clearly most of these individuals are neither diagnosed nor treated for these mood problems (fewer than 6 percent of the general population ever receive treatment for any psychiatric problem).

Kraepelin's descriptions of the symptoms of cyclothymia are lively and vivid:

> These are the people who constantly oscillate hither and thither between the two opposite poles of mood, sometimes "rejoicing to the skies," sometimes "sad as death." Today lively, sparkling, beaming, full of the joy of life, the pleasure of enterprise, and the pressure of activity, after some time they meet us depressed, enervated, ill-humored, in need of rest, and again a few months later they display the old freshness and elasticity.[16]

For many years American psychiatric classification systems regarded cyclothymia as a personality problem. The concept of "temperament," which can be thought of as a person's usual manner of thinking, behaving, or reacting, captures the same idea. Cyclothymia was thought to be better understood as an expression of a person's personality than as an illness caused by an abnormality of brain chemistry. In earlier editions of the *Diagnostic and Statistical Manual* of the American Psychiatric Association (the *DSM*), the disorder was called *cyclothymic personality disorder.* This changed rather recently (in 1980), when *cyclothymic disorder* moved over to the mood-disorder section of the manual—where it remains today.

Individuals with cyclothymic disorder have very frequent ups and downs of mood with only comparatively few periods of "normal" mood. As Kraepelin noted, they seem to "constantly oscillate . . . between the two opposite poles of mood." (This almost constant instability perhaps explains why psychiatrists thought of this as a "personality" characteristic for so long.) As might be expected, constant mood instability causes instability in many areas of the patient's life. In a 1977 study of forty-six patients with cyclothymia, the patients demonstrated a whole variety of oscillations of emotions and behavior—from sleep patterns to work habits to group affiliations.[17]

Cyclothymic disorder begins early in life—in the late teens or early twenties.[18] Although many persons with cyclothymic disorder never develop more severe mood symptoms, a significant number of them eventually have a fully developed depression or manic episode—that is, they develop bipolar disorder. In one study, about 6 percent of patients with cyclothymic disorder eventually had a manic episode, putting them in the bipolar I category, but a higher number (25 percent) developed severe depression—that is, they turned out to have bipolar II.[19] However, perhaps half of patients with the cyclothymic pattern never develop symptoms of full-blown bipolar disorder—a finding that makes cyclothymic disorder a true diagnosis in its own right.

Family-history studies indicate that there is some relationship between cyclothymia and other bipolar disorders. Patients with cyclothymia often have relatives with bipolar disorder but rarely have relatives suffering from depres-

TABLE 2-5 Features of Cyclothymic Disorder

Mood

Frequent alteration between mild depression and mild hypomania
Short irregular cycles (days)
Only short periods of normal mood

Other Features

Patients often wake up with mood changes
Pattern appears in late teens, early twenties
Frequently mistaken for problem with "personality"
Sometimes develops into bipolar I or II

TABLE 2-6 Mood, Thinking, and Behavior Patterns in Forty-six
Cyclothymic Patients

Mood	Percentage of Patients
Irritable periods lasting a few days	50
Explosive, aggressive outbursts	50
Thinking	
Shaky self-esteem alternating between lack of self-confidence and overconfidence	75
Periods of mental confusion alternating with periods of sharpened creative thinking	50
Activity and Behavior	
Increased sleep alternating with decreased need for sleep	75
Unevenness in quantity and quality of work	75
Buying sprees, extravagance, or financial disasters	75
Repeated shifts in work, study, interest, or future plans	50
Drug or alcohol abuse	50
Extroversion alternating with introversion	50
Unexplained promiscuity or extramarital affairs	40
Joining new movement with enthusiasm, rapidly changing to disillusionment	25

Source: Data from H. Akiskal, M. K. Khani, and A. Scott-Strauss, "Cyclothymic Temperamental Disorders," *Psychiatric Clinics of North America* 2 (1979): 527–54, quoted in Frederick K. Goodwin and Kay Redfield Jamison, *Manic-Depressive Illness* (New York: Oxford University Press, 1990), 54.

sions only.[20] As we shall see in chapter 6, treatment experiences seem to confirm this relationship: the mood swings of cyclothymic disorder often respond to many of the same treatment approaches as the bipolar disorders. This finding also confirms that cyclothymia is just as much a "chemical" problem as the other bipolar disorders, and that thinking of the mood swings of cyclothymia as arising from personality problems is not helpful in making treatment decisions.

Bipolar Spectrum Disorders

If you look at the end of the section on bipolar disorders in the fourth edition of the *Diagnostic and Statistical Manual* of the American Psychiatric Association, you will see the category "bipolar disorder not otherwise specified" (also, simply, "bipolar NOS"). This odd category exists because the developers of the *DSM* recognized that there are patients who seem to have *some* kind of bipolar disorder but who don't meet the diagnostic criteria for bipolar I or II or cyclothymia.

Maria is a violinist in the local symphony orchestra. She is nearly sixty but looks much younger. Born in what is now the Czech Republic, she defected to the United States during a tour of a chamber music group in the 1950s. Maria found herself in New York with only a small suitcase of clothes, her violin, and a charming European accent. She credits the latter two with her success in finding good work with several American orchestras over the years.

"I must tell you, Doctor, that my son has started taking lithium and Wellbutrin, just like me. His psychiatrist asked him about my medications and put my son on the same ones. It's so good to know he's being treated by a psychiatrist as brilliant as you."

"Now, now, it was hardly brilliant of me to—"

"Oh, yes, so humble, so modest you are, just like all geniuses."

This was a little game we had played for years, ever since we had come up with a combination of medications that controlled her mood symptoms—for the first time in many years.

Because she had moved to a new city every five years or so, Maria had seen many different professionals for her mood problems—mostly depression. For many of those years she had gotten no treatment at all but simply slogged through her periods of depression on her own. During the 1960s, a physician had given her a prescription for the tranquilizer Valium, and although it hadn't treated her depression very well, it numbed Maria's feelings enough to keep her going. When she moved to a new community, she would be able to get more prescriptions for Valium by reporting to her new doctor that it helped her—which, after a fashion, it did. During the really bad times, Maria used alcohol to augment the Valium's effect. By the time she was in her mid-forties she was well on her way to chemical dependency. One terrible year she lost a job because of missing several rehearsals and an important concert while in a week-long alcohol- and Valium-induced fog during a period of depression. Her husband left her, and a month later she got word that her son, also a talented musician, had dropped out of the prestigious conservatory he had been attending and had disappeared.

Maria's depression worsened to the point that she took a nearly fatal overdose of Valium and alcohol. It was only because the manager of the apartment building where she was living happened to go into her apartment that particular day that she ended up in a hospital rather than in the city morgue. She was eventually admitted to the psychiatric unit for treatment of her depression.

It was in the psychiatric hospital that she started taking an antidepressant for the first time, but the imipramine she was started on made things even worse. Within three days of starting on the antidepressant, Maria started to have manic symptoms. She started staying up all night furiously writing music, convinced that she had discovered new musical forms and new harmonies that would make her fabulously famous and even more fabulously wealthy. Her antidepressant medication was immediately stopped, and she was started on lithium. Within about ten days her mood was back to normal.

On lithium, her depressions were less frequent and less severe, but she continued to have several weeks of low mood every year, and it was during one of these that she had come to see me for the first time. "You were the first doctor to understand that I needed lithium *and* an antidepressant, and that makes you truly brilliant," Maria continued, a raised eyebrow emphasizing her slightly teasing tone.

I was the lucky recipient of a lot of gratitude—gratitude she sometimes archly exaggerated to keep me from taking myself too seriously—because her moods were stable for the first time in years on this combination of pharmaceuticals.

Starting a patient with a history of manic symptoms on an antidepressant is something psychiatric textbooks warn against—but Maria had had manic symptoms only once in her life, at age fifty-three, while taking an antidepressant. Did this really make her bipolar? She didn't have the history of manic or even hypomanic episodes that would make her fit the bipolar I or II diagnosis—yet she clearly had *some* type of bipolar disorder.

Psychiatrists have long recognized that there are many forms of bipolar disorder. Kraepelin noted that "it is fundamentally and practically impossible to keep apart in any way" the various forms of bipolar disorder, and that "everywhere there are transitions."[21] For many years various clinicians have described various types of "soft" bipolar disorder, mostly in patients who came to be treated for depression and whose illness seemed related to bipolar disorder.[22] Terms like *pseudo-unipolar depression* and *bipolar III* have been coined to describe various types of severe depressions that have some features of bipolar disorder but do not fall into traditional categories for bipolar diagnoses. Often these patients have had a long history of depressive-like or manic-like features in their usual mood state, or "temperament," which are punctuated by the more severe mood symptoms that bring them to treatment.

TABLE 2-7 Indicators of "Soft" Bipolar Disorders

Family history of bipolar disorder

History of mania or hypomania caused by treatment with antidepressants

History of "mixed" mood states

Depressive, "hyper," or cycling temperament

Recurrent depressions

As more treatments for bipolar disorder become available and as more research on the mood disorders is done, it is becoming clear that many patients who suffer from mostly depressive symptoms can benefit from treatment with medications for bipolar disorders and may in fact have a type of bipolar disorder.

Nathan is the fifty-five-year-old executive director of a philanthropic foundation. He describes himself as a "workaholic" who for years has worked sixteen- to eighteen-hour days and with only four to six hours of sleep a night. Nathan is famous around town for his buoyant optimism and the boundless energy that he says comes from "making a living giving away other people's money," but his staff knows that he can be impatient and driven when deadlines approach or personnel problems distract him from devoting himself 110 percent to his mission. He came to me for treatment of miserable, irritable, restless feelings that had bothered him for several years but had gotten much worse in the previous few months.

Nathan had had problems with depression before but had never received any treatment with medication. When he was twenty-five he had been depressed after a friend died in a freak accident while both of them were skiing. Nathan had been a graduate student at the time and nearly dropped out of school. When he was in his forties he went through several months of depressed mood, trouble concentrating on his work, and appetite and weight loss that he and his psychiatrist at the time labeled a "midlife crisis" exacerbated by some unpleasant changes in his job. He was in therapy for about three months, and he started feeling better after he embarked on the job search that eventually led to his current position with a prestigious foundation.

"Or maybe it was the other way around," he mused.

"What do you mean?" I asked.

"Maybe I was able to look for a new job because I was feeling better."

"Do you know if other people in your family have had trouble with depression?"

"My father left us when I was three, and they say he was in and out of psychiatric hospitals his whole life. Both his sisters were alcoholics; one committed suicide."

Nathan was proud that despite his childhood in a broken, impoverished home, he now headed a foundation, signed checks for millions of dollars every year, and was courted by presidents of hospitals and universities every day of the week. "So why do I feel this way?" he asked. "It can't just be stress; I thrive on stress. These hopeless feelings come over me, these 'what's the point?' feelings. Why now?"

Nathan suffers from one of the "soft" bipolar disorders that some researchers call *bipolar III*.[23] These patients have a baseline mood that is a bit "higher" than that of most people, a personality characteristic that has been called *hyperthymic temperament*. Their usual energy level is high; they are cheerful, talkative, confident, and sociable. The down side of their personality style is that they tend to become irritated easily and can be impulsive, even reckless at times. They usually have a family history of bipolar disorder and are bothered by recurrent depressions. Antidepressant medication alone can make them more irritable and miserable or provoke a manic or hypomanic episode, but mood stabilizers can be very helpful.

You may have noticed that in this section we have been stretching the disease model a bit by talking about "temperament" and "personality." What is the effect of a person's personality on bipolar disorder and the effect of bipolar disorder on personality? Some persons with serious depressions seem to have a baseline tone to their mood that, while not extreme enough to be called clinical (abnormal), is persistently "up" (*hyperthymic*) or "down" (sometimes called *dysthymic temperament*).

TABLE 2-8 Features of Bipolar III

Family history of bipolar disorder
Hyperthymic temperament:
    Habitual short sleeper—less than six hours per day
    Cheerful, optimistic personality style
    Tendency to become irritable easily
    Extroverted and sociable
Recurrent depressions

While we haven't yet figured out how to classify and accurately diagnose these problems, it is becoming clear that they are related in some way to bipolar disorder, and that many depressed patients who don't seem to have classic "manic-depressive illness" benefit from medications used to treat bipolar disorder.

Rapid-Cycling Bipolar Disorder

Soon after lithium became available for the treatment of bipolar disorder, psychiatrists noticed that some of the sickest bipolar patients didn't seem to derive much benefit from it. These patients clearly suffered from a bipolar mood disorder—they had severe manias and depressions—but they were set apart from other bipolar patients by the frequency of their episodes. Currently, rapid-cycling bipolar disorder is diagnosed if the patient has four or more episodes (mania, hypomania, depression, or mixed state) in one year.[24]

Early impressions and case reports seemed to indicate that there were features other than frequency of episodes that set rapid-cycling bipolar disorder apart from other bipolar disorders. It seemed to occur more often in females, usually began with a depressive episode, and was less responsive to lithium therapy. There also seemed to be some indication that patients with this pattern of illness were more likely to have a history of thyroid gland problems and to have been treated with antidepressant medications.[25] There were suggestions from some researchers that these last two factors—thyroid disease and treatment with antidepressants—might cause "normal" bipolar illness to switch into rapid-cycling illness.[26]

Of these two factors, the most interest has been focused on the possibility that treatment with antidepressant medications can cause the switch from "normal" bipolar disorder into a rapid-cycling form. One study examined the case records of 118 patients who were rapid cyclers (had had four or more episodes of abnormal mood in one year).[27] The researchers found that eighty-six of these patients seemed to have had a change of the course of their illness—that is, they had "switched" into a rapid-cycling pattern. The authors stated that "the majority" of these switched after they were treated with an antidepressant medication.

A more recent study casts some doubt on these findings and on the usefulness of talking about rapid cycling as a specific type of bipolar disorder.[28] In this study, 919 patients were followed over a five-year period, and any who met the criteria for rapid cycling (having had at least one episode of mania or hypomania and three additional episodes of any type during one year) were studied closely for the next five years. Forty-five patients turned out to meet the rapid-cycling criteria, and their family history, treatment course, and course of illness were compared with those of the "normal" bipolar patients.

The picture that emerged from these patients suggested that rapid cycling is a temporary phase of bipolar illness that some patients are prone to—not a particular type of bipolar illness. The rapid cycling stopped after a period of several months in forty-four out of the forty-five patients who were studied. These patients did not have rapid cyclers in their family, although they did have family members with "normal" bipolar illness. The link with thyroid disease and antidepressant treatment seemed weak, and these patients didn't seem any less treatable with lithium than other bipolar patients. As time went on, their rapid cycling gradually stopped. The only finding from the earlier reports that was confirmed was that more women than men had rapid cycling; nearly three-quarters of the patients with rapid cycling were women (bipolar disorder usually affects both sexes about equally).

Some bipolar patients (18.5 percent in this study) seem to go through a period of rapid cycling for some months during which their symptoms are more difficult to control—more women than men (I discuss this in more depth in chapter 14). Although there continues to be suspicion among many clinicians that antidepressant medications can cause some patients to start rapid cycling, the exact causes of rapid cycling remain a mystery, as does, unfortunately, the treatment steps that will prevent it.

Schizoaffective Disorder

Some patients have an illness that has features both of mood disorders and of a very different psychiatric illness: schizophrenia. In addition to mood-disorder symptoms such as depression, hypomania, or mania, these patients have the hallucinations, delusions, and other bizarre mental experiences typical of schizophrenia; they often receive the diagnosis of schizoaffective disorder.

As we have seen in chapter 1, many patients with bipolar disorder develop delusional beliefs or hallucinations. But in the mood disorders, these symptoms can be understood as arising out of the mood state. For example, in a severe depression a patient might have the delusional belief that he or she has a terrible illness like AIDS or has lost all of his or her money, or that family members are being tortured by kidnappers, all beliefs that are—well, depressing. Manic patients may hear the singing of angels or the voice of God—again, hallucinations that can be understood as coming out of the expansive, grandiose mood of mania. Delusions (false beliefs and ideas) and hallucinations (false sensory perceptions such as the hearing of voices) are said to be *mood congruent* when they can be understood as being part of the abnormal mood.

Persons with schizophrenia have bizarre delusions and hallucinations too, but they don't usually seem to bear any relation to a change in mood. Examples of schizophrenic delusions would be the belief that one's next-door neighbors are pumping poisonous gas into one's house, or that one's real spouse and children have been replaced by exact replicas, or that the FBI has implanted a transmitter in one's brain. Patients with schizophrenia sometimes believe that other people are reading their minds or putting into their heads thoughts that are not theirs. They might hear their own thoughts repeated to them aloud or hear the voices of unseen commentators describing their actions to other unseen persons. None of these symptoms has much relationship to mood changes.

When a person has bizarre delusions or hallucinations like those described above or has these kinds of symptoms during times when they do not seem to be in an episode of abnormal mood, the diagnosis of schizoaffective disorder is often made.

What is this disorder, and where does it belong in the classification of psychiatric disease? These are questions that have plagued psychiatry for many years; we still don't have very good answers to them.

Is schizoaffective disorder truly a separate disorder, an illness that shares symptoms with mood disorders and schizophrenia but is neither? If it is, it has been very difficult for researchers to agree on its defining symptoms. In an earlier version of *DSM*, the American Psychiatric Association's classification manual for mental illnesses, the diagnostic category of schizoaffective disorder was included without *any* listing of the symptoms that defined it.

I have seen patients who have been diagnosed with schizoaffective disorder who seem to me instead to have a severe case of a mood disorder that has been difficult to treat. Patients can be delusional and have hallucinations when they are very depressed or very manic, and if they are in a phase of ultra–rapid cycling, these symptoms can change rapidly and do not seem to make much sense in relation to their moods. I have seen patients diagnosed with schizoaffective disorder because they have prominent paranoid symptoms—that is, they believe that they are being watched or followed or talked about. Although paranoid symptoms are very common in some types of schizophrenia and not as common in the mood disorders, close questioning often reveals the mood component in these patients. In a book written during the last century called *A Mind That Found Itself*, Clifford Beers described his battle with a mental illness that was almost certainly bipolar disorder. In one scene he describes a train ride to the psychiatric hospital. As the train passed though the stations along the way, Beers noticed people standing on the station platforms reading the newspaper. He became convinced that they were reading about him. At first glance, this symptom doesn't seem to have any mood component, and in fact it is a rather typical symptom of schizophrenia called an *idea of reference*. Fortunately, however, Beers describes this symptom in great detail in his book and writes that he thought the people on the train platforms were reading about his long history of mental illness and about what a failure he had been. With this added detail—the themes of shame and failure in the symptom—the mood component becomes obvious and the real diagnosis clear: a mood disorder.

Another possible explanation for the mingling of symptoms of a mood disorder and of schizophrenia in one patient is that the patient may suffer from *both* illnesses. If one considers that bipolar I affects about 1 percent of the population and that about 1 percent of the population suffers from schizophrenia, then obviously, if there are no other factors operating to prevent the illnesses from occurring together, as many as 0.01 percent of the population will suffer from both disorders—that is, one in ten thousand. If one adds in other mood disorders such as bipolar II, cyclothymia, and the "soft" bipolar disorders, the numbers of persons with schizophrenia who also have a mood disorder will be even greater. Treatment experience would seem to support this idea: patients with a diagnosis of schizoaffective disorder seem to be most effectively treated with medications for mood disorders used in combination with medications for schizophrenia.

Although someday a treatment that is uniquely effective in schizoaffective disorder may come along and prove my hunch incorrect, I can't help thinking that patients who receive this diagnosis either are very sick bipolar patients or are patients whose combination of symptoms are the result of their having a combination of disorders.

CHAPTER 3

A Summary of the Diagnostic Categories of Bipolar Disorder in *DSM IV*

INDIVIDUALS BEING TREATED BY A MENTAL-HEALTH PROFESSIONAL who read their diagnosis in their medical records or insurance statements often have questions about the diagnostic categories and terms that are used. Psychiatry is one of the few medical specialties that has a more or less official list of disorders and diagnoses, and in this chapter we'll take a closer look at the latest version of this list, the fourth edition of the *Diagnostic and Statistical Manual of Mental Disorders* (the *DSM IV*), developed and published by the American Psychiatric Association. I'll present a brief overview of the *DSM* and explain some of the diagnostic terminology for bipolar disorder.

What Is the *DSM*?

The roots of the *DSM IV* go back at least as far as the United States Census of 1840, which included the category of "idiocy/insanity" in its system for classifying American citizens. By 1880 there were seven categories into which persons with mental illness could be placed: mania, melancholia, monomania, paresis, dementia, dipsomania, and epilepsy.[1] In 1917 the American Medico-Psychological Association—the forerunner of the American Psychiatric Association—developed a statistical manual for use in mental hospitals that included various categories of diagnoses. As time went on other organizations interested in the statistics of mental illness, such as the Veterans Administration and the United States Army, developed their own statistical manuals. After World War II the World Health Association included a long section on mental disorders in the sixth edition of its *International Classification of Disease* (the *ICD 6*).

In 1952 the American Psychiatric Association published the *Diagnostic and Statistical Manual: Mental Disorders* (the *DSM I*), which differed from previous statistical manuals in that it contained a glossary that described the symptoms of the different disorders. Thus, in addition to containing an official list of categories of mental illness, the *DSM I* provided guidance to the clinician in making psychiatric diagnoses. By the time the third edition of the manual appeared in 1980, each category of psychiatric disorders had a list of *diagnostic criteria*—a list of the symptoms and other characteristics of each disorder that were thought to define it and to set it apart from other psychiatric disorders.

As its name now indicates, the *DSM* has become much more than a list of official diagnoses to be used to collect statistics on mental illness; it has developed into a valuable clinical tool, one that has proven immensely useful to clinicians and also to those who do research on psychiatric illnesses. Now, when a patient goes to a new doctor and his or her medical records indicate a diagnosis of, say, "panic disorder" or "anorexia nervosa," the new doctor knows—if the last psychiatrist did his or her job well, of course—that the patient has had certain symptoms and not others, and that the symptoms have troubled the patient for a certain period of time. Use of the *DSM* in research means that when you read a study of some particular psychiatric disorder in a professional journal and read that "the patients met the *DSM IV* diagnostic criteria" for that disorder, you can be sure that the patients all had a certain well-defined collection of symptoms and other characteristics in common, and that the researchers were not mixing, as it were, psychiatric apples and oranges in their study.

Because the *DSM* contains a list of psychiatric diagnoses followed by succinct and clearly written criteria for making those diagnoses, it has the unfortunate effect of making psychiatric diagnosis look easy. It is tempting for individuals who do not have any psychiatric training to regard it as series of symptom checklists that can be easily applied to make the diagnosis of mental illness. Well, why not?

First of all, it is only with an enormous amount of training and experience that one can gain an appreciation for the very wide range of *normal* emotions and behaviors and have a sense of what falls outside this normal range. Significant clinical experience and judgment are needed to decide what constitutes an "expansive mood" or an "increase in energy" that is clinically significant. I have been called to see "manic" patients referred by their counselors or their family members who turn out to be persons simply a bit more intense in manner than most people but whose mood state is perfectly within the normal range. The *DSM* is full of diagnostic criteria that use qualifiers like "clin-

ically significant," "marked impairment," and "excessive involvement in . . . ,"
all requiring judgment based on experience to make a determination. Even
some counseling and therapy professionals, if they have not trained in a setting where they have had the opportunity to see very sick patients, may not really have an appreciation for what constitutes "severe"—simply because they
have never seen and worked with "severely" depressed or manic patients. Non-
professionals will, of course, usually have even less experience with the range
of normal and abnormal moods. Without the experience of seeing many patients with severe mental illnesses and treating them, it is impossible to accurately separate normal from abnormal mental experiences or "clinically significant" mood changes from those that are within the range of the normal.
In psychiatry as perhaps in no other field, the dictum "A little learning is a dangerous thing" holds quite true!

Moreover, as we shall see in chapter 18, many *medical* conditions can
mimic abnormal mood states, dozens of pharmaceuticals can cause depression or euphoric states in some persons, and drugs of abuse can cause all kinds
of moods states and psychoses in almost anyone. Almost all the *DSM* diagnoses contain "exclusion criteria" for medical conditions, such as "the symptoms are not due to a general medical condition." A physician will probably
notice the abnormalities in the facial appearance of a patient with Graves' disease or Cushing's syndrome as soon as the patient walks into the room; the
nonphysician probably has never heard of these illnesses and doesn't know
that they can cause psychiatric symptoms practically identical to those of a
major depression episode. The physician knows well the typical walk of the
patient with Parkinson's disease, the subtle language problems of the patient
who has had a silent stroke—both neurological conditions that can cause
mood symptoms. Obviously, only a clinician trained in the diagnosis and
treatment of physical illness will be able to pick up these sorts of problems.

Finally, just as the range of normal experiences and behaviors is enormous, so is the range (and complexity) of abnormal mental experiences and
behaviors; they cannot be contained in any one book and certainly cannot all
be described in a few dozen diagnostic categories. Another great student of
human behavior, the pioneering researcher on sexuality Alfred Kinsey, once
said, "The world is not divided into sheep and goats . . . Nature rarely deals
with discrete categories. Only the human mind invents categories and tries to
force facts into separated pigeonholes."[2] To paraphrase Kinsey a bit, bipolar
disorder is probably not divided simply into type I and type II, either—and
patients often don't fit into *DSM* pigeonholes.

For these reasons I am not going to list here the *DSM* diagnostic criteria
for the bipolar disorders. I don't want to tempt nonclinicians to engage in self-
diagnosis or diagnosis of family members. The *DSM* is easily available in li-

braries, but it should be considered a reference book for clinicians, not a text-book of psychiatry.

A "Multiaxial" Diagnostic System

A formal *DSM* diagnosis always lists five types of diagnoses and other pieces of clinical information on patients in five separate categories, each of which is called an *axis:*

Axis I	Clinical disorders
Axis II	Personality and intelligence
Axis III	General medical conditions
Axis IV	Psychosocial and environmental problems
Axis V	Assessment of level of functioning

The reason for this complexity is, to put it plainly, that people are complex creatures, and to understand their mental life requires looking at them from several different angles.

Axis I lists the psychiatric illness or condition that is being treated or studied. This is where a mood-disorder diagnosis would go, as would diagnoses like "schizophrenia" or "panic disorder" or "alcohol abuse." This diagnosis will often include additional descriptive terms such as *chronic, acute, severe,* or *recurrent.*

Because symptoms of a mental illness might be expressed differently depending on a person's personality and intellectual ability, these two factors are also recorded in every patient, on axis II. Because these factors will affect how a person copes with a particular psychiatric illness, they are very important in developing plans for treating the disorder. This is also where a diagnosis of a *personality disorder* goes. A personality disorder is diagnosed when patients' personality—a complex mix of temperament, attitudes, and habits, their way of approaching life's problems, their attitudes toward themselves and those around them—causes problems for them in relationships and functioning. For example, persons with *antisocial personality disorder* show a chronic disregard for the rights of others that starts in childhood and continues throughout life. They manipulate and take advantage of others, break the law repeatedly, and show no remorse. This pattern of thinking, relating, and behaving seems to be something ingrained in their personality from an early age rather than the expression of an illness that is imposed upon them at some point. A diagnosis of mental retardation would also be listed on axis II.

Axis III is for any medical problem the individual may have. Examples would be high blood pressure, asthma, kidney failure, or migraine headaches. As we shall see in chapter 18, the axis III diagnosis is sometimes very important in treating a patient with a mood disorder because mood symptoms can be caused or affected by medical conditions such as stroke, Huntington's disease, and thyroid problems, to name only a few.

On axis IV are listed problems in and stresses from the patient's environment that may contribute to his or her difficulties: recent marriage or divorce, job stress or unemployment, chronic poverty, living in an unsafe neighborhood. These factors can also affect how individuals cope with illness as well as their response to treatment. Axis IV information is especially important in the mood disorders, since environmental stressors can be an important precipitating factor for an episode of illness (see chapter 20).

On axis V the clinician records an assessment of the patient's functional level. Using a 1–100 rating scale called the Global Assessment of Functioning (GAF) scale, a judgment is made as to how impaired (or unimpaired) the patient is on the basis of his or her symptoms in everyday life. On this scale, a score of 80 or above means basically normal everyday functioning; below 50 means serious impairment, such as recurrent unemployment due to psychiatric impairments; below 20 pretty much means that the person is in need of psychiatric hospitalization. This axis is perhaps more useful to researchers and statisticians than to clinicians, but it serves to round out a picture of the patient, capturing the person's strengths as opposed to his or her afflictions. For example, an individual might suffer from a severe psychiatric disorder like schizophrenia, have a low IQ, suffer from diabetes, and live at the poverty level but despite all these handicaps be a good parent who contributes to her community; an axis V rating would indicate that despite her psychiatric, intellectual, medical, and environmental problems, this person is functioning rather well. This hypothetical patient's *DSM IV* diagnoses would be as follows:

Axis I	Schizophrenia, paranoid type
Axis II	Mild mental retardation
Axis III	Diabetes
Axis IV	Poverty
Axis V	GAF = 80

Bipolar Categories in *DSM IV*

Only two subtypes of bipolar disorder have been characterized well enough, as to symptoms and course of illness, to have been assigned their own *DSM* categories: *bipolar I* and *bipolar II*. As we saw in chapter 2, in the section on bipolar spectrum disorders, there are probably other forms of the illness that will eventually be described and understood well enough to be demarcated with their own label as well, but for now a patient having another of these "soft" bipolar disorders would be diagnosed with *bipolar disorder not other-*

wise specified (bipolar disorder NOS) according to DSM. Cyclothymic disorder is included in the DSM IV as an axis I diagnosis as well.

For bipolar I patients, the clinician using the DSM is supposed to specify the type of the patient's latest episode, as in "bipolar I disorder, most recent episode manic," or "bipolar I disorder, most recent episode depressed."

The DSM also provides several other descriptive terms called specifiers that can be added to the main diagnosis to describe the current episode better. The clinician can call the episode mild, moderate, or severe. If the patient had not had any episodes in two months, the disorder is said to be in remission (in full remission if there have been no symptoms for two months, in partial remission if there have been only a few symptoms or if the remission has been less than two months).

The specifier with psychotic features can be added if the patient has hallucinations or delusional beliefs (such as those described in chapter 1) during his or her illness. The specifier with catatonic features is added if the patient shows symptoms of catatonia, a rare syndrome in which the patient lies (or sometimes sits or stands) motionless for long periods of time staring into space and has other bizarre physical mannerisms such as rigid posturing, grimacing, or meaninglessly repeating whatever is said to him or her. The specifier with melancholic features can be added when the patient's depressive episode is dominated by loss of ability to experience pleasure (anhedonia), the presence of guilty feelings, a loss of appetite, and the classic daily fluctuation of mood (early-morning awakening with the mood lifting slightly as the day progresses)—in short, the "textbook" depressive syndrome so eloquently described by William Styron in Darkness Visible. Another clinical syndrome, more common in depressive disorders than in bipolar disorders, has been called atypical depression. These patients retain reactivity in their mood (their mood brightens when good things happen); in fact, they seem to have a "hyper-reactive" mood and an especially difficult time with rejection in interpersonal relationships, even when not in an episode of depression. As noted before, this mood syndrome, called depression with atypical features, is not usually seen in bipolar disorder. If the mood episode occurs within four weeks of the birth of a child, it is called depression with postpartum onset.

There is another set of specifiers that describe the course of the illness over time, called longitudinal course specifiers. Bipolar disorders may be with or without full interepisode recovery depending on whether or not patients are completely free of symptoms between episodes.

In chapter 16 we shall learn about a form of bipolar disorder in which patients have repeated depressive episodes occurring regularly in winter and hypomanic or manic symptoms in the summer that has been called seasonal affective disorder. In DSM IV these patients are diagnosed with bipolar I or bipolar II, and the specifier with seasonal pattern is added. Finally, patients

TABLE 3-1 Bipolar Disorders in *DSM IV*

Bipolar disorder I: Mania and depression

Bipolar disorder II: Depression and hypomania

    Severity specifiers for bipolar disorders:
        —mild, moderate, severe (with or without psychotic features)
        —in partial or full remission
    Special syndrome specifiers for bipolar disorders:
        —with catatonic, melancholic, or atypical features
        —with postpartum onset
    Longitudinal course specifiers for bipolar disorders:
        —with or without full interepisode recovery
        —with seasonal pattern
        —with rapid cycling

Bipolar disorder NOS: "Soft" bipolar and bipolar spectrum disorders

Cyclothymic disorder: Depressive symptoms and hypomanias

Substance-induced mood disorder

Mood disorder due to a general medical condition

---

who have had at least four episodes of the disorder in twelve months have a disorder *with rapid cycling.*

When drug intoxication or medical problems mimic manic, hypomanic, or depressive episodes (see chapters 15 and 18), the *DSM* diagnoses *substance-induced mood disorder* or *mood disorder due to a general medical condition* are used. When the mood problem is due to a medical condition, the medical condition and type of mood change are specified in the diagnosis (as in, for example, "mood disorder due to hyperthyroidism, with manic features"). When the problem is due to substance abuse, the type of mood change and whether the symptoms came on during intoxication or withdrawal are specified. (Examples would be "cocaine-induced mood disorder with manic features, onset during intoxication," or "alcohol-induced mood disorder with depressive features, onset during withdrawal.")

CHAPTER 4

The Mood Disease

HAVING REVIEWED THE MANY SYMPTOMS OF BIPOLAR DISORDER AND the many forms the illness can take, I want to take a moment to review just how far we've come in our understanding of this illness—and where we've come *from*. I think that the understanding of any subject is incomplete unless you know a little about its history; and the history of the development of our current thinking about bipolar disorder is not only a fascinating story in its own right but also will provide valuable insights into how psychiatrists think about the diagnostic process and approach the treatment of disorders.

Before "Bipolar"

The ancient Greeks believed that all maladies of mind and body were caused by imbalances among four vital bodily fluids, or "humors." One of the terms we still use to describe depression, *melancholia,* is derived from the Greek word for one of these humors: black bile. According to humoral theory, depression was thought to be caused by an excess of black bile and mania by an excess of yellow bile. In a way this approach to explaining bipolar disorder was remarkably insightful. Modern scientists explaining abnormal mood states might talk of "dysregulation of neurotransmitter systems" rather than too much bile, but the idea that normal physiology is disrupted in the disease still rings true.

Although they were incorrect about the causes of the two opposite mood states of bipolar disorder, several ancient physicians had remarkable insight into the connection between them. Aretaius of Cappadocia (ca. 150) described the syndrome of depression in which patients became "peevish, dispirited, sleepless," and "complain[ed] of life and desire[d] to die." In other patients he described manic symptoms: "At the height of [their] disease [they] have impure dreams, and irresistible desire[s] . . . if roused to anger by admonition or restraint, they become wholly mad." But most remarkably, he stated that "in my opinion, melancholia is without any doubt the beginning and even part of the disorder called mania."[1] Paul of Aegina (625–90) made a similar connection between the two syndromes and based his thinking on humoral theory. Paul also assumed that melancholia was caused by too much ordinary black bile but postulated that mania was caused by an excess of "yellow bile which, by too much heat," had become burned black bile.[2]

Considerations of possible physical causes for the symptoms of bipolar disorder more or less ceased during medieval times, and the symptoms and behaviors that we now recognize as arising from psychiatric conditions were usually attributed to witchcraft or demonic possession rather than to disruptions of a person's physiology. When the Dark Ages gave way to the Renaissance and the Enlightenment, mental illness again became the purview of physicians rather than priests, and modern attempts to understand and classify diseases began. Melancholia and mania were often considered to be two separate disorders by these early physicians. However, a few insightful clinicians, such as the English physician Robert James (1705–76), connected the two syndromes:

> There is an absolute Necessity for reducing Melancholy and Madness [mania] to one Species of Disorder, and consequently considering them in one joint View . . . we find, that they both arise from the same common Cause and Origin, that is, an excessive Congestion of the Blood in the Brain . . . We find that melancholic Patients . . . easily fall into Madness, which, when removed, the Melancholy again discovers itself.[3]

Melancholia and "madness" were thought by most early physicians who wrote about mental disease to predispose to one another, but nevertheless to be entirely different conditions.

It was not until the middle of the nineteenth century that the idea that depression and mania might be expressions of a single mental illness was first proposed. It was proposed by two French *alienists* (a term—from *aliéné*, the French word for "insane"—that was used in France and in English-speaking countries at one time to denote physicians specializing in mental disorders). Jules Baillarger (1809–90) published a paper in 1854 describing an illness he called *la folie à double forme*, and two weeks later Jean-Pierre Falret (1794–1870) rushed a paper into print in the same journal in which he insisted that he had been teaching his students about *la folie circulaire* at the Salpêtrière hospital for ten years. (This was, incidentally, the same hospital where several years later the young Sigmund Freud would begin to formulate his own theories about mental phenomena.) Both men described a mental illness characterized by alternating periods of melancholia and mania that were often separated by periods of normal mood. After the appearance of their original papers, Baillarger and Falret wrote several "me first!" "no, *me* first!" letters to the *Bulletin* of the Imperial Academy of Medicine, each claiming to be the originator of this idea. Which of them deserves credit for being first to describe bipolar disorder is a matter upon which scholars still disagree.[4] But medical historians do *not* disagree about the identity of the psychiatrist who published the first comprehensive description of the mood disorders and established the basis of the classification system for mental illnesses that we still use today.

Dr. Kraepelin and "Manic-Depressive Insanity"

It was the German psychiatrist Emil Kraepelin (1856–1926) who, in 1899, solidified the modern concept of bipolar disorder in the sixth edition of his enormously influential textbook on mental illnesses, *Psychiatrie: Ein Lehrbuch für Studirende und Ärzte.* Kraepelin had been working for several years to develop a logical and comprehensive classification system for major mental illnesses, and successive editions of his *Textbook of Psychiatry* document the development of his thinking.

In the fifth edition he divided severe forms of mental illness into two broad categories: those that had a deteriorating course of illness and those that were "periodic." These two groups are still recognizable in modern classifications of psychiatric disorders, the "deteriorating" group containing the various forms of schizophrenia and related disorders and the "periodic" group containing the mood disorders. Although he was not the first to suggest that mania and depression were both expressions of one disorder, Kraepelin was the first to articulate, clearly and convincingly, the idea that *all* disorders of mood were related to one another:

> Manic-depressive insanity . . . includes on the one hand the whole domain of so-called periodic and circular insanity, on the other hand simple mania, [and] the greater part of the morbid states termed melancholia . . . In the course of the years I have become more and more convinced that all the above-mentioned states only represent manifestations of a single morbid process.[5]

Kraepelin's "manic-depressive synthesis"[6] was a major breakthrough in the understanding and classification of major mental illnesses.

But Kraepelin was more than an academic and theoretician; he was a clin-

FIGURE 4-1 Emil Kraepelin
Source: Hulton Getty Images

ician who saw enormous numbers of patients and recorded his observations of their illnesses in superb detail. As you know from reading them in previous chapters, his descriptions of the symptoms of bipolar disorder are vivid and insightful, and they have really never been surpassed. A former professor once told me that "anyone who thinks they've discovered something new in psychiatry simply hasn't read the German psychiatric literature." I think it's fair to say that anyone who thinks he or she has discovered something new about bipolar disorder—at least, about its symptoms and diagnosis—simply hasn't read Kraepelin.

Kraepelin's contributions, although tremendously significant for those interested in the classification of mental disorders, offered little practical benefit in his time to those afflicted with them. I would imagine that Dr. Kraepelin's patients were more accurately informed about their illness than most patients of that time, and had more reliable prognostic information, but there was really nothing he could do to help them with their symptoms. There was still no treatment for *any* psychiatric condition that offered much hope of alleviating the symptoms or altering the course of the disease. Although the English translation of the chapter on "manic-depressive insanity" in the eighth edition of Kraepelin's textbook is over two hundred pages long, the "Treatment" section is less than five pages long—and most of that consists of warnings about the suicidal behaviors of depressed patients and against discharging them too soon from hospital. In the absence of treatments for manic-depressive illness, patients spent months, even years, in hospitals and asylums.

As the study of mental disorders entered the twentieth century, hopes for more effective treatment of psychiatric disorders rose when scientific discoveries shed some light on the causes of several mental illnesses. In 1906 the German microbiologist August Wassermann discovered a method to detect in human spinal fluid antibodies to the microorganism that causes syphilis. Syphilitic infection of the central nervous system was at the time one of the most common causes of severe psychiatric symptoms, and many patients in mental institutions suffered from "general paresis of the insane," as syphilis with psychiatric manifestations was known. With the development of the Wassermann test, it became possible to diagnose the illness with a very high degree of reliability. For the first time a cause of a form of "madness" had been discovered. That same year another German microbiologist, Paul Ehrlich, developed the first effective treatment for syphilis using arsenic compounds. Although the treatment was crude and dangerous, it was effective enough in the early stages of the disease to reduce the incidence of the illness by 50 percent in several European countries.

We hardly think of syphilis as a mental illness today, but patients with syphilitic infection of the brain can suffer hallucinations, delusions, and mood changes not very different from those seen in bipolar disorder and schizophrenia. An early-twentieth-century psychiatric text describes the mania-like excitement that was sometimes seen in persons with central nervous system syphilis: "The intensity of the excitement is extreme; there is absolute sleeplessness [and] incessant restlessness. The grandiose delusions are the controlling feature of the paretic's thought. The patient . . . comes before us tremulous with emotion, his eye bright, as the overpowering visions of wealth and grandeur float before his mind."[7] The discovery of reliable and effective diagnostic techniques for general paresis of the insane—unfortunately, arsenicals had little effect on the advanced central nervous system disease—was seen by many as an enormous advance in the understanding of psychiatric disorders. Clinicians charged with the care of psychiatric patients had great hopes that the causes of other psychiatric disorders would soon be found.

As more and more powerful microscopes were invented and special tissue stains were developed for brain tissues, various microscopic structures of the brain—the many different types of neurons and the microscopic architecture of the different parts of the brain—became visible for the first time. Anatomical and chemical abnormalities were found to characterize several other diseases with prominent mental symptoms. In 1906 the Swiss neuropathologist Alois Alzheimer discovered abnormal microscopic plaques and tangles of cellular debris in the brains of persons who had died from the progressive brain disease that was eventually named for him. Individuals with *cretinism,* a particularly severe form of mental retardation, were found to have abnormally low levels of thyroid hormones. In 1915 *pellagra,* another mysterious disease, characterized by skin lesions and gradual mental deterioration, was discovered to be caused by a deficiency of vitamin B.

But blood tests and brain studies revealed nothing about manic-depressive illness. Try as they might, pathologists and anatomists could find nothing different or abnormal in the brain structures of individuals with bipolar disorder.

New ways of thinking seemed necessary to understand the mental illnesses for which no physical cause could be found, and shortly after the beginning of the twentieth century, new theories were advanced—by, among others, Sigmund Freud in Europe and Adolf Meyer in the United States—that seemed to have considerable power to explain the basis of these still mysterious illnesses. These theories, boiled down to their essence, held that mental symptoms were reactions to life events in vulnerable individuals—not disease states caused by disruptions in biological functioning. The new theories of mental illness instructed psychiatrists to use "talking cures" to treat their patients.

By carefully exploring patients' biographies in minute detail, physicians attempted to understand what conflicts and life events their patients were re-

FIGURE 4-2 Sigmund Freud
Source: National Library of Medicine

FIGURE 4-3 Adolf Meyer
Source: Alan Mason Chesney Medical Archives and Bachrach Photography

acting to with symptoms of depression or mania. It was the expectation that the proper combination of understanding, reinterpretation, and encouragement could alleviate patients' symptoms. Freud, more than any other early psychiatrist, developed elaborate theories about normal and abnormal childhood psychological development that he felt could explain why some people developed extreme psychological symptoms in response to difficult life situations and events while others did not. Manic-depressive illness and schizophrenia came to be called *functional illnesses* because it was believed that patients with depression or mania or symptoms of schizophrenia had *normal* brain and nervous system functioning. Although Freud and Meyer did not totally discount biological agents as having some role in the causation of these problems, they did not see their patients as suffering from *diseases.* A "functional illness" was believed to be an illness of the mind, not of the brain. These concepts dominated American psychiatry until well into the 1960s.

During these decades most psychiatrists believed that abnormal mental phenomena were caused by traumatic childhood events, poor parenting, repressed sexual feelings, and interpersonal conflicts. They lost interest in the classification and categorization of psychiatric illnesses; the very idea of trying to make a diagnosis in a psychiatric patient seemed a waste of time because the form as well as the cause of a psychiatric problem was as individual as the biography of the patient in whom it occurred. Then in 1949 an unknown Australian psychiatrist published an article in the *Medical Journal of Australia* called "Lithium Salts in the Treatment of Psychotic Excitement."

Dr. Cade and Lithium

By the 1930s and 1940s most physicians interested in the treatment of mental disorders had joined psychoanalytic institutes to learn the theory and practice of psychiatry according to the teachings of Freud and his followers. They trained and practiced mostly in the big cities, mostly treating patients with mild depression or anxiety, patients who had the time, motivation, and money to attend therapy sessions four or five days a week, to explore their past and reinterpret their present in order to become healthier, happier, and better "adjusted." The theories of Freud revolutionized the understanding of many aspects of human behavior, and they continue to form the basis for the practice of psychotherapy. But there were many patients who benefited little from these new ideas. They were the patients Dr. Kraepelin had cared for: the victims of schizophrenia and manic-depressive illness.

For these patients, housed for months or years in (mostly public) hospitals and asylums, the therapeutic armamentarium had not changed much in two hundred years: bed rest for the depressed; physical restraint for the agitated; baths, tranquilization with morphine and bromides, and the use of a number of other substances thought to have beneficial effects, among them quinine and even cod-liver oil. None of these interventions had any but the most insignificant effects on serious mental illness.

John F. J. Cade, M.D., senior medical officer in the Mental Hygiene Department of Victoria, Australia, was convinced that manic-depressive illness was a biological disorder, not a psychological one. Working in his laboratory to determine if some toxin might be present in the urine of patients with manic-depressive illness, Cade became especially interested in urea and uric acid, by-products of protein metabolism found in urine, and was testing the toxicity of these compounds by injecting small amounts of them into guinea pigs.

One of the technical problems with this work was that uric acid is rather insoluble in water, making preparation of injectable solutions difficult at higher concentrations. Looking for a soluble urate salt to use instead of uric acid, Cade consulted prior research and discovered that uric acid was easiest to dissolve in water when it was combined with a lithium ion as lithium urate. He injected small amounts of lithium urate into the guinea pigs and noticed that uric acid seemed to be much less toxic in this form. This suggested to Cade that the lithium component of the compound might have some sort of protective effect against urate toxicity. To determine what the effect of the lithium ion might be, he injected lithium carbonate—the carbonate ion is a harmless compound found in things such as baking soda—and discovered that "after a latent period of about two hours the animals, although fully conscious, became extremely lethargic and unresponsive to stimuli for one to two hours before once again becoming normally active."[8]

Cade admits in his original paper that "it may seem a long distance from lethargy in guinea pigs to excitement in psychotics," but asylum doctors of the time were desperate for new treatment possibilities, so Cade decided to administer lithium preparations to several patients who were chronically agitated. The effect on patients with mania was dramatic:

> Case I—W.B., a male aged fifty-one years, who had been in a state of chronic manic excitement for five years, restless, dirty, destructive, mischievous and interfering, had long been regarded as the most troublesome patient in the ward. His response was highly gratifying. From the start of treatment on March 29, 1948, with lithium citrate he steadily settled down and in three weeks was enjoying the unaccustomed surroundings of the convalescent ward. As he had been ill so long and confined to a "chronic ward," he found normal surroundings and liberty of movement strange at first. He remained perfectly well and left the hospital on indefinite leave with instructions to take a dose of lithium carbonate, five grains, twice a day. He was soon back working at his old job. However, he became more lackadaisical about his medicine and finally ceased taking it. His relatives reported that he had not taken any for at least six weeks prior to his readmission on January 30, 1949 and was becoming steadily more irritable and erratic. On readmission to the hospital he was at once started on lithium carbonate, ten grains three time a day, and in a fortnight had again settled down to normal. He is now (February 28, 1949) ready to return to home and work.

> Case VIII—W.M., a man of fifty years, was suffering from an attack of recurrent mania, the first of which he had had at the age of twenty. The present attack had lasted two months and showed no signs of abating. He was garrulous, euphoric, restless and unkempt when he started taking lithium. Two days later he was reported to be quieter. By the ninth day he was definitely settling down and the following day commenced work in the garden. By the end of two weeks he was practically normal—quiet, tidy, rational, with insight into his previous condition. This was in marked contrast to his condition a fortnight before when he had to be locked in a single room at night . . . and was too restless to eat in the dining room owing to his unsettling effect on the other patients.[9]

Dr. Cade had treated ten manic patients with lithium, and all ten had shown the same dramatic improvement. He had also given lithium to six patients with "dementia praecox" (schizophrenia) and three patients with "chronic depressive psychoses," but with less effect. The agitated patients with schizophrenia became less agitated but had "no fundamental improvement"; the depressed patients had "no improvement."

It is often emphasized in textbooks and articles on the history of lithium treatment that Cade's discovery of lithium's efficacy in bipolar disorder was pure accident—an observation that misses an important point. Cade, like many hospital psychiatrists, but unlike perhaps many other psychiatrists of his time, was pursuing a biological intervention for what he believed was a biological disorder. His case descriptions reveal that even though he had little specific therapy to offer them, he had taken a complete history of his patients' course of illness, carefully examined them, and, following in the footsteps of Emil Kraepelin, made a *diagnosis* based on his examination and history taking. Cade's approach to these severely ill patients—his assumption that they suffered from diseases rather than from emotional reactions—provided the theoretical underpinning that made his discovery possible. A psychiatrist who believed in "reactions" and "functional illness" would have been unlikely to divide patients into the diagnostic categories of mania, schizophrenia, and depressive psychosis and report on differential efficacy of a pharmaceutical in each group (let alone have been looking for toxins in the urine of patients with mania).

One would think that the news of Cade's discovery would have spread like wildfire. It did not. In fact it was several decades before lithium was approved for the treatment of bipolar disorder by the United States Food and Drug Administration. Why this incredible delay?

Part of the reason was the state of world psychiatry following the end of World War II. German psychiatry was in ruins, literally and figuratively. The German psychiatric establishment, which had produced superb clinicians like Kraepelin and Freud and many other pioneers in the science of mental disorders, had been mesmerized by the Nazi movement. Prominent German psychiatrists had enthusiastically participated in the expulsion of Jewish colleagues from the profession and in the murder of the patients they had been charged to care for. Thousands of mentally retarded and mentally ill individuals were gassed in the years leading up to the war and during the war. When Cade wrote of his work with lithium, Germany was no longer providing leaders in psychiatric medicine; rather, German psychiatry was in dire need of rehabilitation.[10]

In the United States and England, psychoanalytic theories had replaced the traditional medical practices of evaluation, diagnosis, and treatment with the prescription of the "talking cure" for all emotional problems. Accurate psychiatric diagnosis simply didn't exist; any patient with severe symptomatology was usually called "schizophrenic" and admitted to a state psychiatric hospital for little more than custodial care. Ronald Fieve, the American psychiatrist who would champion the use of lithium in the United States in the 1970s and who was instrumental in getting American psychiatrists to prescribe it for their patients, observed that during the late 1940s and the 1950s in New York, he "rarely met with the diagnosis of manic-depression . . . It had virtually disappeared. Most cases of excitable, talkative, and elated behavior were being diagnosed as schizophrenia."[11]

But a Danish psychiatrist, Morgans Schou, realized that Cade's discovery represented a real breakthrough, noting in a 1954 paper that "it is rather astonishing that [Cade's] observation has failed to arouse greater general interest among psychiatrists."[12] Schou and his colleagues did the careful clinical trials that eventually resulted in the development of recommended dosages and preparations of lithium for the treatment of symptoms of bipolar disorder. Perhaps more than any other clinical researcher, Schou established the efficacy of lithium treatment for mania. Even more important was his discovery of lithium's ability to *prevent* the reoccurrence of symptoms in patients with bipolar disorder.

In 1957 another breakthrough occurred in the treatment of mood disorders when Roland Kuhn, a Swiss psychiatrist, discovered that a compound originally developed as an antihistamine had remarkable therapeutic effects on depressed patients. He reported his results in a Swiss medical journal in a paper reprinted the next year in English as "The Treatment of Depressive States with G 22355 (Imipramine Hydrochloride)." But Kuhn also noticed that in some patients imipramine simply replaced one mood problem with another: "In marked manic-depressive psychosis, i.e., if the depressions are easily and frequently replaced by manic-like phases or actual manic states, the reaction is less favorable . . . the tendency arises for the depression to switch over into a manic phase."[13]

In one of their first papers on the use of lithium in manic patients, Schou and his colleagues had pointed out that "the beneficial effect of lithium in cases of mania appears to offer new possibilities for a study of the *pathophysiology* of the manic-depressive psychoses."[14] The discovery of the therapeutic effects of imipramine on depressed patients and the observation that it could precipitate mania in patients with "manic-depressive psychosis" were two more clues that bipolar disorder might be more than a psychological "reaction."

The fact that a chemical (lithium) made the symptoms of mania go away indicated that mania had at least some biochemical basis. The discovery of the different effects of imipramine on depressed persons with and without a history of mania reinforced the disease model for bipolar disorder. Persons with a history of mania became manic if they took imipramine; persons who did not have a history of mania (usually) did not. Imipramine was not simply a "manio-genic" drug, a drug that produced euphoria in everyone who took it. The fact that only bipolar individuals became manic from it suggested that their illness had a different biochemical basis from depression. The distinction between *bipolar* and *unipolar* depressions became established in psychiatric diagnosis. The modern age of psychiatry had begun, as had the search for more and better pharmaceutical treatments and for the physical basis of these disorders.

PART II

TREATMENT

Several years ago I heard a classical guitarist being interviewed on the radio. He said that he was often asked by strangers, usually people who didn't know much about classical music, whether he played the *electric* or the *acoustic* guitar. "I hate that term, *acoustic guitar*. I'd rather just say I played the guitar," he said. "But after the electric guitar was invented, I suppose somebody had to come up with a term for a nonelectric guitar."

There is a term for psychiatric problems that many nonpsychiatrists use that I dislike, and that's *chemical imbalance*. It's a term that we started hearing used in the 1970s to describe psychiatric problems that were not psychological reactions or "functional" problems (as I described them in chapter 4) but rather were illnesses caused by some malfunction of brain physiology. To paraphrase the guitarist, I suppose somebody had to invent a term for psychiatric illnesses as opposed to purely psychological conditions, but *chemical imbalance* implies several things about psychiatric illnesses that are very misleading.

First is the idea that all disturbances of mental life fall into two mutually exclusive categories: "chemical" and "nonchemical" (or perhaps "chemical" and "psychological" might work better). As we shall see in this next group of chapters, such a division is not possible, for the "chemical" and "psychological" aspects of mental life interact and overlap in many ways. Second, to say that a psychiatric problem like bipolar disorder is simply an "imbalance" of brain chemicals is a monumental oversimplification of what really lies at the root of these problems. The fantastically complex human brain is not simply a cantaloupe-sized organ bathed in a soup of "chemicals" that can be adjusted by the addition of medications to achieve a "balance" (as a chef adds a little more salt or another pinch of cayenne to make a favorite recipe come out right).

In the first chapter in this part of the book I'll do my best to explain what causes bipolar disorder (without using the term *chemical imbalance*) and also touch on how we think the medications used to treat the illness work. The details here are a bit complicated, but the basics are not difficult to grasp. This chapter might require a slower, more careful reading pace for those unfamiliar with terms like *neurotransmitters*, but this effort will pay off later, allowing you to understand the use of medications in bipolar disorder much better.

Then we'll start talking about treatment more specifically, beginning with a review of the pharmaceuticals used in the treatment of the disorder. We'll also cover electroconvulsive therapy—still a very valuable resource for the treatment of mood syndromes—and, last but certainly not least, the important role of counseling and psychotherapy in the treatment of the illness. We'll end with a brief overview of the treatment approaches and some principles of treatment that I think are important to remember.

CHAPTER 5

The Brain: Neurons, Neurotransmitters, and More

IN ORDER TO UNDERSTAND THE TREATMENT OF BIPOLAR DISORDER, you have to know a little bit about how the brain works. In this chapter I'm going to give you a brief overview of the functioning of the human nervous system, just enough to help you understand a little bit about how psychiatric medications work.

A number of years ago the psychiatrist and neuroscientist Nancy Andreasen wrote a book about the new discoveries in biological psychiatry.[1] The title—*The Broken Brain*—makes the point that psychiatric illnesses like bipolar disorder and schizophrenia are caused by biological and chemical malfunctions of the brain, not repressed memories or traumatic childhoods. Although we still don't know exactly what these malfunctions are, we are getting very close to understanding some of the biological mechanisms that might be involved. In this overview of brain functioning, I want to tell you about what scientists think might be "broken" in bipolar disorder.

Many people imagine that the human brain is a kind of wonderful computer. Although this is a vast oversimplification of the true capabilities of the brain, it's a good place to start in trying to understand how this fantastic organ of the mind works.

Like the computer that I'm using to write these words, a human brain receives input, processes the information it receives, and then delivers output. Like a computer, it stores information and often uses this stored information to help process the input it receives. The brain receives its input from the sense

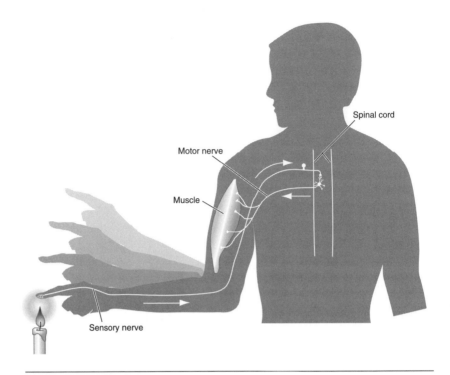

FIGURE 5-1 Spinal reflex

organs—the eyes, ears, taste buds, touch receptors, and so forth—and delivers output in terms of behavior.

The simplest example of this input-processing-output circuit in our nervous system is the spinal reflex. This circuit, so simple and so automatic in its operation, deserves its label: *reflex*, meaning a simple behavior that requires no "thinking" to be effectively carried out. If you inadvertently touch the hot surface of a stove or an open flame, a nerve ending detects the resulting tissue damage and fires a message up the fingertip through your hand and arm along a nerve fiber (called a *sensory* nerve) that ends in the spinal cord. Here the first nerve communicates with another nerve, which dispatches a message down again through another fiber (a *motor* fiber, so called because it causes movement) to activate the arm muscles to pull the finger back from the source of the heat. If you've ever actually had this experience, you may have noticed that your hand pulled away before you even felt the pain. This is because the brain, where consciousness resides, is not even involved. (The message that is eventually sent up to the brain from the level of the spinal cord with the pain signal is more or less an "FYI" message that will be stored in the memory system. This painful memory will almost certainly lessen the chances of the same thing happening again!)

Let's look at a more complicated example of the input-processing-output circuit, one that is not just a reflex (or at least not, perhaps, as reflex as it should be). Say you're walking down the street and pass a florist's shop that has a sign in the window saying, "Don't forget, next Sunday is Mother's Day!" You realize with a start that you *have* forgotten, so you march into the shop, pull out your credit card, and order some flowers for Mom. Same process, really: input (seeing the sign), processing (Yikes! I forgot!), and output (pulling out that trusty plastic). There are many more steps, and some very complex ones, this time around: seeing the sign, using the language functions of the brain to draw meaning from those little shapes we call letters that are on the sign, drawing on memories of what is expected of one on Mother's Day, an emotional tone generated by the feelings you have for your mother that affects the process—I could go on and on. There is a complex interaction of many, many nervous system functions, some very simple (the posture reflexes that let you walk into the shop without falling flat on your face are nearly as simple as the spinal reflex example above) and others more complex (the arithmetic functions that allow you to answer the question, How big an arrangement can I buy without going over my credit limit?). Obviously no computer built today is capable of anything approaching as complex a processing task as this. Why not?

You may know that a computer computes by means of many thousands of microscopic switches embedded into its processing chip. Information is stored via the pattern of "on" and "off" in the switches and is processed via the flow of input signal through these switches. The human brain contains about eleven billion nerve cells or neurons—but as powerful as a computer with eleven billion switches might be, the brain is many orders of magnitude more impressive than that. This is because the neuron is not just a switch that is either "on" or "off," but rather is an impressive microprocessor in its own right. Each neuron receives input from many other neurons, processes this information, and sends output to many others. The brain, then, is not like a computer with billions of switches; it is more like a network of billions of computers, all capable of being individually programmed. Each neuron in the brain may receive input and transmit signals to up to fifty thousand other neurons. The number of *all* the possible connections in the human brain is incomprehensibly large, a hyper-astronomical number on the order of the number of molecules in the universe! (So even if we could figure out how to build such a computer, there would be no place on the planet big enough to put it.)

I'm going to jump the gun a little and tell you now that there is a lot of evidence that bipolar disorder is a defect in the mechanisms by which the individual neurons are programmed and reprogrammed. But before we get to that, we need to talk about *neurotransmitters*.

Although the human nervous system uses electrical signals to do much

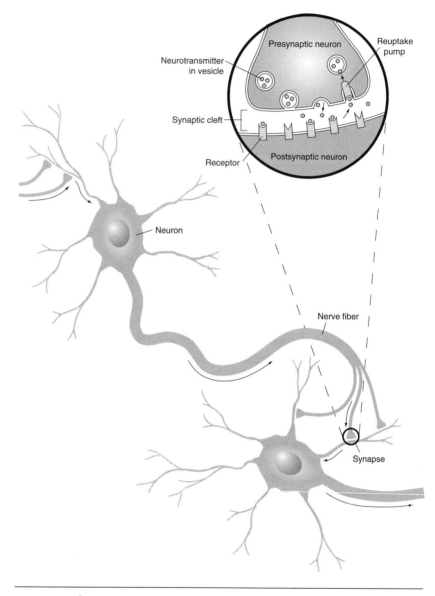

FIGURE 5-2 Synapse

of its work, it uses chemical signals called neurotransmitters as well. Let's go back for a moment to the spinal reflex to examine how these signals do their jobs. Remember that in this reflex a pain signal from the finger travels up a nerve fiber into the spinal cord. As you might guess, this is an *electrical* signal, a change in the electrical charge of the nerve fiber that travels as a pulse along its length until it reaches a cell body that resides in the spinal cord. This cell body is like one of the eleven billion tiny computers I mentioned earlier, except that it is in the spinal cord, not in the brain. When enough pain signals come in, this microscopic CPU starts communicating with the motor nerve responsible for pulling away the finger, and when the motor neuron computes that it is necessary, it fires its own pulse of electrical energy down the motor nerve to the muscles. The signals by which the two neurons communicate with each other are the chemical ones I mentioned: molecules called neurotransmitters.

The neurons send these chemical signals to each other at a site called the *synapse,* an area where the two neurons nearly touch, separated only by an ultramicroscopic space called the *synaptic cleft.* The first neuron (the *presynaptic neuron*) releases packets of neurotransmitters, which flow across the narrow synaptic cleft and link up with targets called *receptors* on the next cell (the *postsynaptic neuron*), with the neurotransmitter molecules fitting into their receptors as keys fit into locks. There needs to be some mechanism for this signaling system to be turned off and reset, of course. After a pulse of neurotransmitter molecules links up with receptors across the synapse, they must somehow be removed in preparation for the next pulse. This happens in a variety of ways in different cells, but one of the most important mechanisms is a *reuptake* into the cell that released them. There is a reuptake pump on the presynaptic neuron that removes neurotransmitter molecules from the synapse and takes them into the interior of the cell, where they are repackaged for rerelease.

There is a constant level of neurotransmitter release across the synapse, a steady tone of chemical signal that pulses up at times. The neurons are not just "switches" that can only be set to "on" or "off" but rather tiny information-processing units that are constantly communicating with other neurons to which they are functionally linked.

Now let's turn to mood disorders again. What is "broken" in these illnesses? As you will see, much of what we know about the biological and chemical basis of mood disorders was discovered *after* an effective medication had been accidentally discovered. In a backwards kind of investigative process, by figuring out where in the brain these medications are active and what they do to brain chemistry—and usually we determine this by observing the effects of these pharmaceuticals on brain preparations in test tubes—we have discovered clues about the location and function of the "broken" mechanisms in mood disorders.

It wasn't long after Ronald Kuhn discovered that G 22355 (imipramine) was an effective antidepressant that someone started to look at the effect of this pharmaceutical on brain chemistry. It was discovered that imipramine was a powerful inhibitor of the reuptake of a group of neurotransmitters called *neurogenic amines* (or *neuroamines*), the most important one being *norepinephrine*.

Remember that neurons turn off their chemical signals ("turn *down*" is probably more accurate) by scooping up neurotransmitter molecules from the synapse and repackaging them. Just as partially closing the drain in a bathtub will cause the tub to begin to fill with water, if you block the reuptake of neurotransmitter molecules, the net effect will be an *increase* of neurotransmitters in the synapse. This observation—that antidepressants increased the amount of neurotransmitters in the synapse by blocking their reuptake—led to the "amine hypothesis" of the mood disorders. This theory basically stated that depression was caused by an abnormally low level of norepinephrine and mania by too high a level. (This may be where the unfortunate term *chemical imbalance* had its origins.)

But further work soon indicated that this was too simplistic an explanation. As more antidepressant medications were discovered, it was found that some very effective ones seemed to have little effect on the norepinephrine system. Fluoxetine (Prozac) is one of a family of pharmaceuticals that are powerful inhibitors of the reuptake of another neurotransmitter, called *serotonin*, but they have very little direct effect on norepinephrine. Some antidepressants also seem to affect other neurotransmitters too, especially one called *dopamine*. As a result of these discoveries, the amine hypothesis was revised, and it was proposed that mood was regulated by a complex interplay of *several* chemical circuits in the brain. It is now thought that this interplay of activity among *all* these systems is disrupted in depression and in mania.

Another argument against a simplistic theory involving too much or too little norepinephrine is an observation about the time course of the antidepressant-induced chemical changes in the brain. Antidepressant-induced changes in neurotransmitter levels at the synapse occur almost *immediately* after the drug is taken—in a matter of hours. But it takes several *weeks* for these agents to start alleviating the symptoms of depression. If the problem were simply too little neurotransmitter in the synapses of certain brain circuits, why would it take several weeks after the drug raised transmitter levels at the synapse for the symptoms of depression to get better? It has been suggested that the neurons respond to these higher levels of neurotransmitters by changing their receptor molecules, either making them more sensitive to the neurotransmitters or putting more of them in the synapse. The idea is that antidepressants work by triggering an "up-regulation" of receptor sensitivity in the neuron. This hypothesis continues to be popular among neuroscientists interested in the chemistry of mood disorders.

This theory fits nicely with some of the work done on the chemical mapping of the brain. Several nuclei of cells deep in the brain that use norepinephrine as their neurotransmitter project a vast network of fibers that terminate on sheets of cells contained on the convoluted surface of the brain, the *cerebral cortex.* This area of the human brain, thought to be responsible for many of our most complex "higher" brain functions, is rich in cells with receptors for norepinephrine. This system seems to be ideally organized to affect the tone of functioning of the entire cerebral cortex—making it a good candidate for the target system of antidepressants. There are serotonin pathways that originate deep in the brain and project widely across the cortex too, and pathways that use other neurotransmitters as well. The balance of activity among these different systems and their interaction with each other are probably very important in the regulation of mood. These neurotransmitter systems are probably where antidepressant medications do their work.

Because of its unique therapeutic effects in bipolar disorder, there has naturally been a lot of effort to figure out where lithium is active in the brain and what its effect on brain chemistry is. In fact, the investigation of lithium's effect on brain chemistry is leading scientists closer than ever to the probable "broken" mechanism in bipolar disorder.

Lithium doesn't seem to affect neuroamine levels anything like antidepressants do, and it doesn't interact with neuroamine receptors or the reuptake pumps. In fact, it doesn't have any of the types of direct effect on cells that the antidepressants do. It has only been in the last few years that the probable site of lithium action has been found, and it's not at the synapse at all. Lithium—and perhaps the newer mood stabilizers as well—seems to work at a different cellular level: *inside* the neuron.

Although the precise fit between a neurotransmitter and its receptor molecule has often been compared to the precise fit of a key into a lock, it has become apparent that the receptor is much more than just a lock. Starting in the 1970s, scientists were able for the first time to elucidate the structure of cellular receptors and discover the details of these complex and elegant mechanisms. Receptors on the surface of the cell are coupled with structures called *G proteins* that extend through the cell membrane and link up with a complex array of other proteins and enzymes that help regulate various functions of the cell. The G proteins act as transducers, converting data from outside the cell (the presence or absence of the receptor molecules) into functional changes inside the cell. They don't do this directly but rather by a complex cascade of chemical events that probably also includes turning genes located inside the cell on and off.

There is evidence that lithium has direct effects on G proteins, but scientists have recently started to focus on several other groups of molecules that work inside the cell as "second messengers." The neurotransmitters—molecules that bring messages from other cells to the neuron—are considered the *first* messengers. The *second* messengers are molecules that are *inside* the cells

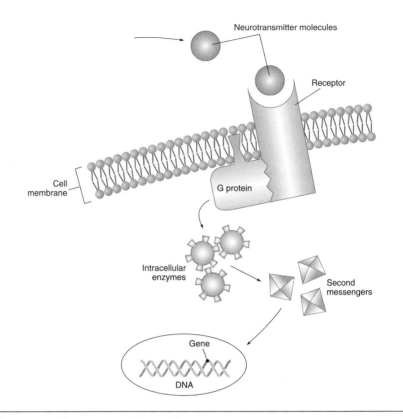

FIGURE 5-3 Receptors and G proteins

and are activated by G proteins to travel within the neuron to set various cellular switches in the cell membrane (the covering of the neuron) and in the main control center of the neuron (the nucleus). Several lines of evidence support the alternative idea that lithium acts by inhibiting enzymes responsible for the manufacture of several second-messenger molecules.

You can think of the G protein/second-messenger system as a communications and activity-monitoring system for the neuron, constantly assessing the level of neurotransmitter activity and, perhaps by turning genes on and off, constantly altering and adjusting the functioning of the neuron in response to this activity. This is the "programming and reprogramming" of the neurons discussed earlier in the chapter. This process might be a necessary part of maintaining mood within a normal range. This system might control mood by somehow "tuning" the responsiveness of our mood state to experiences and environment. Perhaps bipolar disorder is the result of a broken G protein/second-messenger system of neurons in the norepinephrine and serotonin circuits that regulate mood: the system's sensitivity is incorrectly tuned too high or too low, and abnormal changes of mood result. This might explain why the highs and lows of bipolar disorder are *both* effectively treated by lithium. Perhaps the lithium ion fits into and stabilizes the shape of one of the component molecules of this system, or in some other way helps this system to work better and do its job more effectively, thus stabilizing mood.

This idea may also explain why antidepressants help with symptoms of mood disorders (including bipolar disorder) and take several weeks to do so. Antidepressants may artificially raise the amounts of neurotransmitter in the synapse to very high levels, high enough that even a "broken" G protein/second-messenger system can respond, turning on genes that start making receptor molecules or other cell components necessary to retune the neuron, a process that takes several weeks.

It may be a while before we understand how all the molecular and cellular pieces of this complicated story fit together, but the work to unravel the basic cause (or causes) of bipolar disorder is proceeding very rapidly. And when we understand exactly what is "broken" in bipolar disorder, the job of fixing it will become much easier.

CHAPTER 6

Mood-Stabilizing Medications

MOOD STABILIZERS ARE MEDICATIONS THAT HAVE BOTH ANTIMANIC and antidepressant effects. Perhaps an even more important effect of this class of medications is their ability to decrease the frequency and severity of episodes of the illness. Thus, the vast majority of patients with bipolar disorder are treated with one or another of these medications, and sometimes with several.

Lithium

We've already learned about the discovery of the therapeutic effects of lithium in bipolar disorder by John Cade in the 1940s. But lithium has an even older history as a pharmaceutical that is just as interesting as the story of Dr. Cade and his guinea pigs. In the second century A.D. the Greek physician Seranus Ephisios recommended that physicians treating patients suffering from mania should prescribe "natural waters, such as [from] alkaline springs."[1] We now know that the water from many alkaline springs is rich in lithium. Roman physicians recommended that their patients "take the waters" at various springs for a number of physical and mental ailments. Down through the centuries centers for healing grew up around natural springs all over Europe, from the little town in eastern Belgium called Spa to Bath in England, Wiesbaden in Germany, and dozens of other towns in Italy and Greece. As the science of analytic chemistry developed, curious chemists and physicians evaluated these various springs and found that the waters of many were rich in lithium.

In the middle of the nineteenth century, lithium compounds were tried as treatments for gout and kidney stones. Gout is a painful arthritic condition caused by abnormally high levels of uric acid in the body; the uric acid is deposited in the form of urate crystals in the joints and other tissues. Kidney stones are also usually made up of urate compounds. It was hoped that lithium would somehow dissolve the urate crystals in the joints of gout patients as well as urate kidney stones. (Remember that Dr. Cade picked lithium urate to work with because it is the most soluble of the urate compounds.) Unfortunately lithium did not turn out to be helpful for these problems, and the approach was abandoned. But this work led to the formulation of pharmaceutical preparations of lithium compounds and to information on the range of safe doses for lithium preparations in humans.

In the late 1940s lithium came to medical attention again when lithium chloride was introduced as a salt substitute for patients with medical problems, like heart disease and high blood pressure, that required them to be on a low-sodium diet. But when heart patients were given salt shakers full of lithium salts to sprinkle on their food, the results were catastrophic for some. Because lithium is toxic in surprisingly low concentrations, substituting lithium chloride for sodium chloride turned out to be a disaster. There were many reports of severe lithium poisoning and even several deaths among these patients. The use of lithium as a salt substitute ended. This episode had the effect of giving lithium a very bad reputation among physicians, and it was perhaps another factor that explains the delay in the acceptance of Cade's discovery of lithium's efficacy in bipolar disorder.

In the 1950s the Danish psychiatrist Morgans Schou began what was to be his life work: the development and refinement of the therapeutic use of lithium for the treatment of bipolar disorder. Schou very quickly became convinced of the effectiveness of lithium in treating acute mania, and he was one of the first clinical researchers to become convinced of another therapeutic effect of the drug: its ability to prevent further episodes of illness (lithium's preventative or *prophylactic* effect). Schou had a more difficult time convincing his colleagues around the world that lithium could prevent recurrences of bipolar disorder, and that patients should take it even after their acute symptoms had subsided. In 1967 Schou and his colleague Paul Christian Baalstrup reported on eighty-eight patients who had taken lithium for several years and who had a dramatic reduction in the frequency and duration of their mood episodes. Several patients who had been sick for several weeks out of every year experienced a complete remission of their illness that lasted for over five years; their illness had essentially stopped.[2]

As they treated more and more patients with the medication, it became so apparent to Schou and his colleagues that lithium favorably altered the course of bipolar illness that they had ethical qualms about doing a more rig-

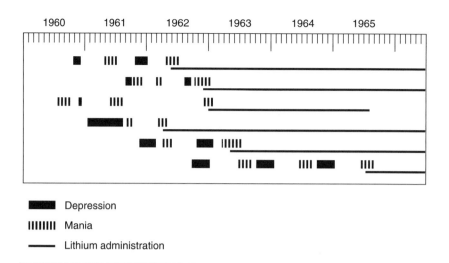

FIGURE 6-1 This graph illustrates data from six patients in Baalstrup and Schou's early study on the prophylactic effects of lithium on bipolar symptoms. Each line represents the symptom course of one patient. In all these patients, when lithium was started, episodes of mania and depression stopped completely.

Source: Data from Paul Baalstrup and Morgans Schou, "Lithium as a Prophylactic Agent: Its Effect against Recurrent Depressions and Manic-Depressive Psychosis," *Archives of General Psychiatry* 16, no. 2 (1967): 162–72.

orous placebo-controlled study—one in which bipolar patients would be divided into two groups, some to receive lithium and the others a placebo. In a rather cranky 1968 article titled "Prophylactic Lithium: Another Therapeutic Myth?" several British psychiatrists scolded the Danes for reporting their results without a placebo group.[3] So Baalstrup and Schou did a lithium discontinuation study in which they took patients who had been stable on lithium for at least a year, divided them into two roughly equal groups, and in one group substituted a placebo for the lithium.

This was a *double-blind study,* the most powerful type of clinical trial possible—and now pretty much a required test for new medications. In this type of study, patients who are similar as to age, diagnosis, severity of illness, and so forth and who agree to be in the study are divided into two groups. One group gets the medication that is being tested, and the other group (the *control* group) gets a placebo (or in some studies the control group receives a standard medication for the disorder being studied). The patients do not know whether they are taking the new medication or the placebo, and neither do the clinicians who examine them for improvement; hence the term *double*-blind. It is only after the trial is over that the group membership of the patients is re-

TABLE 6-1 Therapeutic Profile of Lithium

Medication class:	Mood stabilizer
Brand names:	Eskalith, Eskalith CR
	Lithobid
	Lithonate
	Lithotabs
Half-life:	14–30 hours
Metabolism:	None
Elimination:	Kidneys
Birth control:	Probably mandatory
Other considerations:	Blood levels extremely important

vealed and the results of the two groups compared. Improvement is measured objectively by using checklists of symptoms and various rating severity scales that have been verified as being reliable and valid.

The results of the Baalstrup and Schou study were dramatic: of the thirty-nine patients whose lithium was replaced with the placebo, twenty-one relapsed within five months; of the forty-five other patients, those whose lithium was not replaced, *none* had a relapse. In 1970 Baalstrup and Schou published their results in the same British journal in which their critics' paper had appeared,[4] establishing once and for all that lithium's prophylactic effect on bipolar disorder was no myth.

THERAPEUTIC PROFILE

It has now been shown in many more studies that lithium is not only effective in the treatment of acute mania and acute bipolar depression but also that it reduces the severity, duration, and frequency of manic and depressive episodes of bipolar patients.

Lithium is a naturally occurring element found in mineral springs, seawater, and certain ores. Like its close cousin sodium, it is never found in its pure form in nature but only combined with other ions as a salt of one type or another. It is mined on an industrial scale for use in the manufacture of ceramics and batteries. Therapeutic lithium preparations usually contain lithium carbonate (the carbonate ion combined with lithium; when the carbonate ion is combined with the closely related sodium, it forms sodium carbonate, which is common baking soda).

Because it is an element, lithium is not chemically transformed (metabolized) within the body, and because lithium atoms are so similar to sodium atoms, the body handles lithium in much the same way it handles sodium. Lithium is rapidly absorbed through the gastrointestinal tract, enters the bloodstream, and is eliminated from the body by being filtered out by the kidneys.

Descriptions of the effects of a pharmaceutical in the body always include one vital statistic: the medication's *half-life*. This is a measure of how quickly the body gets rid of a pharmaceutical. Specifically, it is the time required for half the amount of the drug to be eliminated or metabolized by the body. Put another way, it is the time it takes for the body to reduce the level of the medication by half. The half-life of lithium in adults is between fourteen and thirty hours.[5] Another useful number that can be derived from the half-life statistic for any medication is the time it takes for the level of medication to build up to a constant level in the body, or in other words the time it takes for the amount being taken in to equal the amount being eliminated: the *equilibrium point*. By a series of mathematical steps that we don't need to detail here, it can be shown that the equilibrium point is always the same for all medications: five half-lives. This means that since the half-life of lithium is roughly one day, it will take roughly five days for a patient who starts on lithium to reach a steady level of lithium in the bloodstream. It also means that if the lithium dose is changed, it will take about five days for the blood level to stabilize at the new level.

Because of the toxicity and even deaths that were reported when heart patients sprinkled it freely on their food as a salt substitute, there was a significant delay in the acceptance of lithium as a therapeutic agent. Lithium is a powerful pharmaceutical, one that must be treated with respect. It has a very low *therapeutic index*, meaning that the difference between the therapeutic dose and a toxic dose is small.[6] Fortunately, lithium can be measured in the bloodstream accurately and fairly cheaply, and the dosage adjusted according to the results.

It is important to pay attention to lithium blood levels not only to prevent toxicity but also because it has been clearly demonstrated in clinical studies that lithium needs to be present in the bloodstream at a certain level to be effective in most patients. (We speak of a "therapeutic level" in discussing the effective range of lithium in the bloodstream for treatment, not a "normal level." Lithium is a trace element in the body, normally present in undetectable concentrations. Bipolar disorder is not a lithium deficiency!) Just what that level should be has been a matter of debate, and the definition has shifted over the years. But an important study from Massachusetts General Hospital found that a level of between 0.8 and 1.0 meq/L (this stands for milliequivalent per liter and is a chemical measure of concentration) was most effective.[7] In this double-blind study, bipolar patients were divided into two groups, a "standard-dose" group, whose lithium levels were kept between 0.8 and 1.0 meq/L, and a "low-dose" group, whose levels were maintained between 0.4 and 0.6

TABLE 6-2 Comparison of Higher and Lower Lithium Levels in Relapse Rates of Bipolar Disorder

Treatment Group	Any Relapse	Depressed	Manic/ Mixed	Hypomanic	Withdrew from Study
Standard range (0.8–1.0 meq/L)	6 (12%)	3 (6%)	3 (6%)	0	24 (51%)
Low range (0.4–0.6 meq/L)	21 (44%)	1 (2%)	17 (36%)	3 (6%)	11 (23%)

Source: Data from Alan Gelenberg, John Kane, Martin Keller, Phillip Lavori, Jerrold Rosenbaum, Karyl Cole, and Janet Lavelle, "Comparison of Standard and Low Levels of Lithium for Maintenance Treatment of Bipolar Disorder," *New England Journal of Medicine* 321, no. 22 (1989): 1489–93.

meq/L. The researchers found that the relapse rate in the "low-dose" group was more than double that in the "standard-dose" group.

There's more to these data than may initially meet the eye, however. Many more patients from the "standard-dose" group than from the "low-dose" group dropped out of the study because of side effects. The take-home message seems to be that levels closer to 1.0 meq/L are more protective—but that many people have trouble taking that high a dose because of side effects. Many psychiatrists compromise and try to maintain their patients at levels between the "standard" and the "low" range. Dr. Schou, whom many consider to be the father of lithium therapy, has recommended levels of 0.5 to 0.8 meq/L.[8] However, it's very clear that some people have good control of their symptoms on even lower levels—elderly patients, for example. Lithium levels thus need to be individualized to the patient, and Dr. Schou also points out that "changes in lithium levels as small as 0.1 to 0.2 [meq/L], upward or downward, may substantially improve patients' quality of life during maintenance treatment."[9]

The lithium level in the bloodstream rises after every dose, peaks in about two hours, then begins to fall again. If a patient takes his or her lithium two or three times a day, there will be several peaks and valleys. Because the level is rising and falling throughout the day, it is important that the blood be drawn at a time when it can be correctly interpreted. The convention that has been adopted is to use a twelve-hour level, making it convenient to draw blood in the mornings. For most patients this means getting to the lab twelve hours after their bedtime dose—for example, at 11 A.M. if the bedtime dose was taken at 11 P.M. the night before—with their usual morning dose in their pocket or purse.

TABLE 6-3 Treatable Side Effects of Lithium

Side Effect	Remedy
Nausea, diarrhea	Take immediately after meals
	Switch preparations
Weight gain	Diet and exercise
Thirst, frequent urination	Diuretics may help, but *must* be prescribed by an M.D. (see text)
Tremor	Beta-blocker medications
Flareup of preexisting dermatologic conditions	Dermatologic preparations
Hypothyroidism	Thyroid medications

SIDE EFFECTS

Individuals vary widely in their sensitivity to the side effects of lithium (and to all medications, for that matter). Some patients will have none, others will have several. Fortunately, almost all the side effects of lithium can be eliminated or managed.

Many of lithium's side effects are *dose-related*, meaning that the higher the dose, the more severe the side effect. One side-effect management strategy, then, is simply to lower the lithium dose. The advantages of higher levels are clear, as noted above, but most physicians will try to maintain patients at the lowest possible dose that controls their symptoms.

Because of its similarity to sodium, lithium has some of the same effects that an increased intake of sodium (salt) would have: increased thirst, increased urination, and water retention. These side effects are often temporary and subside as the body adjusts to the medication. If they do not, the judicious use of medications that promote urination and excretion of excess body water (diuretics) can help. However, *do not take diuretics without consulting your physician!* Some diuretics have the effect of raising lithium levels and can cause severe lithium toxicity. The lithium dose must usually be lowered by half, and lithium blood levels must be scrupulously monitored. There have been reports of persistent and severe increased urination—diabetes insipidus, which has nothing to do, incidentally, with diabetes mellitus, the common "sugar diabetes"—that progresses over time. A few cases of impaired kidney functioning have also been reported. Both these problems are rare and slow to develop. Nevertheless, in addition to monitoring lithium blood levels, blood tests that measure kidney functioning are routinely ordered for patients taking lithium.

Lithium is irritating to the gastrointestinal tract and can cause nausea or diarrhea. Taking it on a full stomach can ease these problems considerably. A fine shaking in the hands (tremor) can occur at higher levels. Medications used to treat tremors, called *beta blockers,* are frequently prescribed and can be very helpful. Weight gain can be a very annoying side effect and unfortunately has an equally annoying remedy: diet and exercise.

Between 5 and 35 percent of patients treated with lithium develop depression of thyroid gland functioning (hypothyroidism).[10] When hypothyroidism develops, it seems to be able to cause an increase in mood cycling in addition to the symptoms of too little thyroid hormone (low energy, dry skin, sensitivity to heat, and puffiness around the eyes are some of the early signs). If a person's lithium seems to "stop working"—that is, if the person suddenly seems to have an acceleration in his or her illness—the development of hypothyroidism should be suspected. When it does occur, hypothyroidism can be treated by thyroid replacement medications. A test of thyroid functioning is the third in the battery of blood tests routinely ordered for lithium patients.

Lithium can cause flareups of preexisting skin conditions but only rarely causes the onset of new dermatological problems. Patients with psoriasis, acne, and other dermatological problems may need closer follow-up from their dermatologist.

Lithium has been associated with birth defects. Remember that by the time a woman misses her period after conceiving, development of many of the embryo's major organs is already well on its way. Stopping a medication after a woman *knows* she is pregnant may well be too late to prevent a birth defect. Women of childbearing age should practice birth control while taking lithium if there is any chance of becoming pregnant. Lithium is secreted in breast milk, and patients taking lithium should not breast-feed. (See chapter 14 for a more complete discussion of medications and pregnancy.)

Another side effect that troubles a significant number of patients taking lithium is a noticeable dulling of mental functioning and coordination. Patients complain that their ability to memorize and learn is affected, and that they have a difficult-to-explain sense of mental sluggishness. For years these complaints were downplayed by clinicians, many of whom tossed them off as coming from patients who simply weren't used to feeling "normal," who missed the mental alacrity of hypomania. This view seemed to be supported by research using psychological tests on bipolar patients taking lithium, research that has been basically inconclusive. But when nonpatient volunteers were administered lithium and similarly tested, there was a small but definite drop-off in their performance, proving that lithium-induced mental sluggishness is a very real problem for some patients.[11] This is a dose-related side effect and is another reason to strive for the lowest possible maintenance dose of lithium that still controls mood symptoms adequately. Fortunately these problems also often get better with time.

Valproate (Depakote)

The development of valproate (brand names include Depakote and Depakene) for the treatment of bipolar disorder is another convoluted study in serendipity. Valproic acid is a carbon compound similar to a number of others that are found in animal fats and vegetable oils: a fatty acid. It was first synthesized in 1882 and was used for many years as an organic solvent for a variety of purposes. (Remember that a solvent is a liquid that other substances easily dissolve into.) Many decades ago pharmacists used it as a solvent for bismuth salts, which were used to treat stomach and skin disorders.

In the early 1960s scientists looking for treatments for epilepsy were working with a group of new pharmaceutical compounds that appeared promising but were difficult to dissolve. (Is this beginning to sound familiar?) They discovered that valproic acid was an effective solvent for the compounds they were testing, and they started using it to dissolve their test drugs for animal experimentation. As they tested their various new pharmaceuticals, the results they obtained seemed to be confusing—until someone realized that it didn't matter *which* of the new pharmaceuticals was used. As long as *any* of them was dissolved in valproic acid, the drug was found to be effective in stopping epileptic seizure activity. It soon became obvious that it was the valproic acid that was stopping the seizures, not what was dissolved in it. By 1978 valproate had been approved by the Food and Drug Administration for use in treating epilepsy.[12]

In the 1960s there were some reports that valproate might be helpful in treating mood disorders, and throughout the late 1960s and early 1970s a French psychiatrist named Lambert published a series of papers about using it to treat bipolar disorders. After the discovery that another antiepilepsy medication, carbamazepine, was effective in treating mania (we'll cover this story in the next section of this chapter), interest in the possibilities of valproate as a mood stabilizer grew. In the mid-1980s several studies by American psychiatrists of the use of valproate in treating bipolar disorder appeared, and ten years later valproate had become firmly established as an effective antimanic medication and a mood stabilizer.

Valproate's therapeutic action in bipolar disorder—or in epilepsy, for that matter—is still completely unknown. It is known to improve neuronal transmission in the brain that is mediated by the neurotransmitter gamma amino butyric acid (GABA). GABA seems to have an inhibitory or modulating effect on many brain circuits, and valproate's effect may be to enhance this modulator in some way.

Valproate has been established to be effective in the treatment of acute mania. It also appears to be effective in preventing the recurrence of, and to reduce the severity of, episodes of bipolar disorder. Its effectiveness in the treatment of acute depressive episodes of bipolar disorder has been less impressive.

In reading about this medication, you may become confused by the many names it goes by: valproate, valproic acid, divalproex sodium, not to mention the brand names Depakote and Depakene. Many chemicals, many medications included, consist of two parts called ions, one of which is positively charged and the other negatively charged. When the two parts exist together as a *compound,* the charges cancel each other out and the system is stable. Valproate is actually the name of the ion. When it is associated with a hydrogen atom, the result is valproic acid. In combination with a sodium ion, it becomes sodium valproate. Depakote is a preparation manufactured by Abbott Laboratories consisting of a stable combination of sodium valproate and valproic acid that is called divalproex sodium. Depakene is Abbott's brand name for its valproic acid preparation.

The half-life of valproate is between six and sixteen hours in adults.[13] Thus, it reaches equilibrium in the body more quickly than lithium, in two to three days. Valproate seems to have a number of advantages over lithium in the treatment of acute manic episodes. First, it appears to work more quickly. Whereas lithium may take up to three weeks to have its full effect, valproate has been shown to start working within five days, especially if a "loading-dose" strategy is used.[14] This strategy consists of calculating a valproate dose (based on a patient's weight) that should cause the patient to reach a therapeutic blood level and then starting at that dose immediately; this differs from the usual practice of beginning with a lower "starting dose" that is gradually raised. This method of treating acute mania has been reported to be highly ef-

TABLE 6-4 Therapeutic Profile of Valproate

Medication class:	Mood stabilizer (anticonvulsant)
Brand names:	Depakene, Depakote
Half-life:	6–16 hours
Metabolism:	Affected by other antiepilepsy drugs
Elimination:	Liver
Birth control:	Probably mandatory
Other considerations:	Blood levels helpful; blood tests for liver inflammation are needed

fective, well tolerated in many patients, and very fast acting.[15] Valproate also seems to be more effective than lithium for certain subgroups of manic patients: patients with rapid cycling (four or more mood episodes per year) and patients with mixed mania (a mixture of manic hyperactivity and pressured thinking with depressed or unpleasant mood).[16] Valproate is much less toxic than lithium.

One big disadvantage of valproate is that it does not seem to be as helpful in acute depression as lithium is. Neither is it very effective in preventing recurrences of depression.[17] This suggests that valproate may be a better choice for patients with rapid cycling or with mixed mania, but that patients with classic euphoric mania and major depressions may have better control of their symptoms with lithium.[18]

Like lithium, valproate can be measured in the bloodstream; unfortunately, it is more difficult to measure, and the test is therefore more expensive to perform. Blood levels above 45 mcg/ml (micrograms per milliliter) have been shown to be necessary for the therapeutic effect to occur, and side effects become more problematic at levels greater than 125 mcg/ml.[19] Several studies show that valproate is helpful in cyclothymia, bipolar II, and "soft" bipolar disorders, and that lower doses and lower blood levels are required than in the treatment of bipolar I with valproate.[20] As with lithium, blood for valproate levels should be drawn twelve hours after the last dose of medication.

SIDE EFFECTS

Valproate has a milder side-effect profile than lithium and is not nearly as toxic in overdose. Side effects that are common as a patient starts taking the medication include stomach upset and some sleepiness. These problems usually go away quickly. Increased appetite and weight gain have been reported, though in my own experience this is an uncommon problem. Mild tremor occurs as well and can be treated with beta-blocker medication. A few patients report hair loss, usually temporary, which resolves even more quickly with vitamin preparations containing the minerals zinc and selenium.[21]

Several cases of severe liver problems have been reported in patients taking valproate, but these have occurred almost exclusively in children taking the drug for control of epilepsy, most of whom had other medical problems and were taking several different medications. A 1989 review article states that no fatalities from liver problems caused by valproate had ever been reported in patients over the age of ten who were taking only valproate. Just to be on the safe side, however, a blood test that can detect liver inflammation is done on patients taking valproate for the first time and is repeated at appropriate intervals while they are taking it. Since valproate can also in rare cases cause a drop in blood counts, a complete blood count is usually done as well. These are very rare problems, and even when they do occur, they develop slowly and usually during the first six months of therapy. Thus, they can be picked up with routine blood tests. Nevertheless, patients on valproate should be on the lookout for signs of liver or blood count problems, which include unusual bleeding and bruising, jaundice (yellowing of the eyes and skin), fever, and water retention.

Valproate has been associated with birth defects, and as with lithium, women in childbearing years should practice birth control while taking valproate if there is any possibility of becoming pregnant.

Carbamazepine (Tegretol)

After the introduction of carbamazepine (brand names include Tegretol and Epitol) for the control of epilepsy in the 1960s, several reports appeared indicating that epilepsy patients taking carbamazepine who also had mood problems not only had good control of their seizures but had improvement in their psychiatric symptoms as well. It was a small step then to test carbamazepine in patients with mood problems who did not suffer from epilepsy. Much of the earlier work on the use of carbamazepine in bipolar disorder was done by Japanese clinicians looking for an alternative to lithium, which was not approved for use in Japan until years after it was available in the United States. In 1980 a study appeared in the *American Journal of Psychiatry* titled "Carbamazepine in Manic-Depressive Illness: A New Treatment,"[22] and the race was on to refine the use of this medication in bipolar disorder and define the group or groups of patients it helped the most.

THERAPEUTIC PROFILE

Every once in a while a patient of mine requests that he or she be prescribed the "best" mood stabilizer or antidepressant medication there is. I usually respond by telling the person that if there were a "best" medication in a particular class of medications, it would be the only pharmaceutical manufactured and prescribed. What would be the point of using anything else? The reason there are so many drugs of a particular type is that some work better or have fewer side effects in individual patients. Many newer medications don't seem to be more effective than available ones when studied in large groups of patients, but they are clearly better for certain patients who can't take or don't respond to an older agent. (This point sometimes seems lost on some HMOs and other health-care organizations that try to keep their physicians from prescribing more expensive new medications instead of older, less expensive ones and justify their policies on the basis of studies of *groups* of patients that make the older medications look "just as good" as newer ones—but that's another story altogether.)

Carbamazepine is one of these medications that don't seem to have any advantage in most studies of groups of patients but that work very well—in fact, work when other medications do not—in some patients. In one well-designed double-blind study, manic patients who took carbamazepine actually seemed to do worse than patients taking lithium.[23] But most psychiatrists have had a patient like "Ms. B.," whose case history was reported in a paper from the National Institutes of Mental Health in 1983:

> Ms. B., a 53-year-old woman, had a history of treatment resistant, rapid cycling manic-depressive illness that required continuous state hospitalization from 1956 to her admission to NIMH in 1978. She had been non-responsive to [antipsychotic medications, tricyclic antidepressants] and lithium . . . After institution of carbamazepine, both mood phases improved dramatically and she was able to be discharged . . . During a subsequent hospitalization her severe mania again did not respond to [antipsychotic medications] and she was not able to leave the hospital until she was treated with carbamazepine.[24]

In this study the authors noted that "additional improvement appeared to occur when [antipsychotic medications] were used in conjunction with carbamazepine or when lithium and carbamazepine were used in combination." This has become carbamazepine's niche, a second-line mood-stabilizing agent used in patients who do not respond to other agents, and often used in combination with other agents.

Like the other mood-stabilizing medications, carbamazepine can be measured in the bloodstream, and blood levels can be used to adjust the dose. Unfortunately not much work has been done on carbamazepine blood levels in bipolar patients, so the therapeutic range used for the treatment of epilepsy is usually the target psychiatrists aim for in their patients.

Carbamazepine is metabolized in the liver, and like some other drugs it causes the liver to increase the level of the enzymes that metabolize it. This means that the longer a person takes carbamazepine, the better the liver be-

TABLE 6-5 Therapeutic Profile of Carbamazepine

Medication class:	Mood stabilizer (anticonvulsant)
Brand names:	Epitol, Tegretol
Half-life:	18–55 hours (shortens after time)
Metabolism:	Complex; affects and is affected by other drugs
Elimination:	Liver
Birth control:	Probably mandatory
Other considerations:	Blood levels helpful; blood tests for liver inflammation and blood abnormalities needed

comes at getting rid of it. So after a few weeks the blood levels may go down, and the dose may need to be increased. This increase in liver enzymes can also affect other medications the patient might be taking, including certain tranquilizers, certain antidepressants, other epilepsy medications, and some hormones, including birth control preparations. It is very important that all physicians involved in a person's care know when carbamazepine has been started so that dosage adjustments can be made.

SIDE EFFECTS

Carbamazepine can cause the sort of general side effects that many medications affecting the brain can cause: sleepiness, lightheadedness, and some initial nausea. These problems tend to be short-lived and dose-related.

As with valproate, there have been rare cases of liver problems associated with carbamazepine, so blood tests for liver inflammation are routinely done. There have been even rarer reports of dangerous changes in blood counts, so blood cell counts are also done, especially in the first several weeks of therapy. Some cases of a rare but dangerous skin reaction called Stevens-Johnson syndrome have occurred. Although all these problems are very, very rare, patients should be on the watch for the development of a rash, jaundice, water retention, bleeding or bruising, or signs of infection.

Lamotrigine (Lamictal)

Lamotrigine (brand name Lamictal) is another antiseizure medication that appears to have therapeutic effects in patients with bipolar disorder. Studies began to appear in the 1980s showing that it was a useful "add-on" therapy in epilepsy patients already taking other antiseizure medications. During the early investigations of this use, researchers noted that patients who took lamotrigine for seizure control reported an improvement in their mood and sense of well-being—even if it hadn't helped much with their seizures. Lamotrigine has several effects on the brain that might explain its efficacy in bipolar disorder. It appears to inhibit release of the neurotransmitter glutamate, an amino acid that causes stimulation of various neural circuits. Lamotrigine is also thought to affect at least one of the same second-messenger systems that lithium affects, the inositol triphosphate system.[25]

THERAPEUTIC PROFILE

Because it is such a new agent, lamotrigine's place in the treatment of bipolar disorder is still unclear. The most exciting aspect of its profile is its apparent effectiveness in bipolar depression. One of the first reports on its use in the treatment of bipolar disorder described a patient who had suffered from rapid-cycling bipolar I disorder since the age of fourteen.[26] In the year before

TABLE 6-6 Therapeutic Profile of Lamotrigine

Medication class:	Mood stabilizer (anticonvulsant)
Brand names:	Lamictal
Half-life:	15–24 hours
Metabolism:	Affected by carbamazepine, valproate
Elimination:	Liver
Birth control:	Recommended
Other considerations:	Rarely causes severe skin rashes, but has good side-effect profile

starting lamotrigine, he had been either depressed or manic continuously, with no period of normal mood. When he was first seen by the research team, he had been severely depressed and had not responded to lithium or carbamazepine or an antidepressant. On lamotrigine his depression symptoms gradually improved, and eleven months later he hadn't had a recurrence of either depressive or manic symptoms.

Other studies indicate that lamotrigine works well with other mood stabilizers in treatment-resistant patients and can sometimes turn a partial medication response into a more complete one.[27] Lamotrigine is a welcome addition to the present array of mood stabilizers—especially in light of its apparent antidepressant effects.

Lamotrigine has a half-life of fifteen to twenty-four hours, and its metabolism is affected by taking carbamazepine and valproate. Blood levels are not routinely ordered for lamotrigine because of its low toxicity and because therapeutic effects have not been correlated with a particular blood level range.

SIDE EFFECTS

Aside from some initial nausea or gastrointestinal upset and the sort of side effects that many medications affecting the brain can cause—sleepiness, lightheadedness or dizziness, headache—lamotrigine has a very good side-effect profile. The most serious side effects that have been reported are a very dangerous type of skin rash called Stevens-Johnson syndrome and toxic epidermal necrosis (this problem is much more common in children than in adults, and for that reason lamotrigine is not prescribed to patients under the age of sixteen). Patients should examine their skin carefully, especially during the first several weeks of therapy, and stop the medication and get in touch with their doctor at any sign of skin rash.

Other Mood Stabilizers

A number of other agents show promise for the treatment of bipolar disorder. For the most part the promise of these medications is based on a few case reports of a therapeutic effect, or in some cases they are medications in the same class as other pharmaceuticals already shown to be helpful.

Gabapentin is yet another antiseizure medication that seems to be a mood stabilizer as well. As with the others, reports of beneficial effects on mood-disorder symptoms in patients in whom it was being used to treat epilepsy came first, and a few indicators of effect in bipolar disorder followed. One case report concerned a man with bipolar disorder who had refused to take lithium and who had liver disease and low blood counts caused by alcoholism.[28] Since he wouldn't take lithium and his medical problems made use of valproate or carbamazepine risky, he was tried on gabapentin. He had a "dramatic" decrease in manic symptoms, his sleep pattern returned to normal, and best of all he reported no side effects. Another preliminary study gave gabapentin to twenty-eight patients with various forms of bipolar disorder who had not had a satisfactory response to lithium, valproate, or carbamazepine.[29] Eighteen of the twenty-eight had a positive response. Gabapentin is not metabolized in the liver and so does not affect the blood levels of other medications; it doesn't need blood level monitoring, and it has a very good side-effect profile. It remains to be seen whether or not gabapentin will live up to these encouraging early reports.

Other antiepilepsy drugs that have attracted the interest of clinical researchers on bipolar disorder are *topiramate* and *tiagabine.* Ongoing research may result in these drugs also being introduced as mood-stabilizing medications.

CHAPTER 7

Antidepressant Medications

ANTIDEPRESSANT MEDICATIONS ARE HIGHLY EFFECTIVE IN TREATING the depression of bipolar disorder. They must be used carefully and judiciously, however, because these medications can push a bipolar patient from a depression into a manic state and cause other problems as well. In fact, the observation of manic symptoms in patients being treated for tuberculosis with a medication called iproniazid led to the development of the class of antidepressant medications called monoamine oxidase inhibitors (MAOIs).

Despite these findings and the risks associated with antidepressants in persons with bipolar illness, antidepressant medications have become very important in the treatment of bipolar disorder. Many patients will take an antidepressant, at least temporarily, for symptoms of bipolar depression.

Tricyclic Antidepressants (TCAs)

Although tricyclics are now infrequently used as antidepressants, our discussion starts with this group because they were the first antidepressant medications developed, and because they still provide the standard by which all promising new pharmaceuticals for the treatment of depression are judged.

They are called tricyclics because of the three rings that can be seen in their chemical structure (see figure 7-1). Although some of them have an effect on serotonin systems in the brain, the primary effect of the tricyclics in the brain seems to be an inhibition of reuptake of the neurotransmitter *norepinephrine* by neurons. Remember that reuptake of neurotransmitters into the neuron

• HCl

CHCH$_2$CH$_2$N(CH$_3$)$_2$

AMITRIPTYLINE

CH$_2$CH$_2$CH$_2$N(CH$_3$)$_2$

IMIPRAMINE

FIGURE 7-1 Chemical structure of two tricyclic antidepressants, showing their characteristic three-ringed structure

after they have been released into the synaptic cleft and done their work signaling the next cell is the means by which the synapse is "reset." Norepinephrine is usually removed quickly from the synapse and pumped back into the cell that released it in order to turn off and reset the system. By blocking the removal of norepinephrine, these medications seem to prolong or intensify the norepinephrine's message to the cell in some way.

The discovery of this effect of tricyclics on norepinephrine in neurons was one of the first chemical effects of a medication active in the brain measured in the laboratory. The observation that tricyclics *increased* the amount of norepinephrine in the synapse, along with the discovery that certain other medications used to treat high blood pressure *reduced* norepinephrine—and were observed to cause depression in some patients—led to the early amine hypothesis of the mood disorders: the theory that depression was caused by too little norepinephrine and mania, presumably, by too much. However, further testing indicated that tricyclics increased amines in the synapse within *hours* of taking them, whereas the therapeutic effect of antidepressants was known to take several *weeks* to occur. This led to a search for alternative explanations to the amine hypothesis.

When it was discovered that tricyclics cause a change in the number and sensitivity of norepinephrine receptors on the postsynaptic neuron, it was suggested that this "down-regulation" of the norepinephrine system by tricyclics was the sought-after therapeutic effect of these medications. But other newer antidepressants don't have this down-regulating effect on norepinephrine.

The fundamental biochemical effect of antidepressants that is actually responsible for their benefits still remains a mystery. It is thought that the change in neuroamine signaling at the synapse that antidepressants cause may set off a cascade of events involving second-messenger systems that eventually results in the improvement of the symptoms of depression. Unfortunately the answer to the question, How do these medications work? remains largely unknown.

Tricyclics have become such an infrequently prescribed group of antidepressant medications principally because of their many side effects. As with all medications, some patients can take these medications easily and without unpleasant side effects, but many patients have to put up with a few side effects in order to get the benefits. Fortunately the side effects are all dose-related, and most are temporary.

You may remember that Ronald Kuhn found imipramine, the first tricyclic, among a group of compounds that had some antihistamine effects. It's not surprising, then, that these medications affect some people the way antihistamines do, causing mild sleepiness and sometimes what some of my patients have called a "weird" or "spacey" feeling for the first day or two after starting on them. Tricyclics block another neurotransmitter called acetylcholine, which is used in the division of the nervous system that regulates many "automatic" functions of the body such as digestion. These *anticholinergic* side effects include a slowing down of the gastrointestinal tract causing constipation and dry mouth. The focusing of the lens of the eye and the emptying of the urinary bladder are also controlled by this system, and tricyclics can cause blurry vision and urination difficulties also, though usually only in high doses. Patients with a history of glaucoma or urinary tract problems

TABLE 7-1 Tricyclic Antidepressants

Pharmaceutical Name	Brand Name	Usual Dose (mg/day)	Sedation	Anticholinergic Side Effects*	Weight Gain
Amitriptyline	Elavil	100–200	+++	+++	++
Amoxapine	Ascendin	200–300	+	+	+
Clomipramine	Anafranil	100–200	++	+++	+
Desipramine	Norpramin	100–200	−/+	+	+
Doxepin	Sinequan	100–200	+++	++	++
Imipramine	Tofranil	100–200	+++	++	++
Maprotiline	Ludiomil	100–150	++	++	++
Nortriptyline	Pamelor	75–150	+	+	+
Protriptyline	Vivactil	15–40	−/+	+	+

*Anticholinergic side effects include dry mouth, constipation, and blurred vision.

should be monitored closely by their physician while taking these medications. Tricyclics also cause weight gain in many patients.

Tricyclic overdoses are very dangerous and are responsible for many of the completed suicides by overdose in people with mood disorders. Although the lethal overdose is up to twenty times the normal dose for an adult, children are more sensitive to the toxic effects of these medications, and just a handful of tablets can be fatal in a small child. For this reason these medications must be scrupulously safeguarded in households with children.

Selective Serotonin Reuptake Inhibitors (SSRIs)

It will come as no surprise that a new pharmaceutical that had none of the tricyclic side effects listed above and was not toxic in overdose caused something of a sensation when it was introduced in 1988. That pharmaceutical was fluoxetine (Prozac), and *sensation* sums up the response to this medication nicely.

For a time it seemed that everyone you talked to was either taking Prozac or reading *Listening to Prozac* (or *Talking Back to Prozac,* or *Prozac Nation*). A Prozac capsule showed up on the covers of *Newsweek* and *New York* magazines, and the drug was featured in innumerable other magazines and newspaper articles. Prozac was a miracle drug that was going to change the world.

The inevitable backlash took about another year to get going, but once it did, psychiatrists couldn't pay their patients to take Prozac. Full-page ads denouncing the drug ran for weeks in *USA Today,* and various talk-show hosts found people who gladly came on national television to swear that Prozac had made their lives miserable.

Fortunately all that nonsense is over now, and the (rather boring) facts have emerged. Prozac and the similar pharmaceuticals that have come along since are as effective as the tricyclics are as antidepressants—they may even be *more* effective in some people—and they have a vastly superior side-effect profile.

Unlike the tricyclics, this new class of antidepressants has little direct effect on norepinephrine in the brain but instead blocks the reuptake of another neurotransmitter into neurons, another amine compound called serotonin. The very potent and specific serotonin reuptake blockade effects of these agents give this class its name: *selective serotonin reuptake inhibitors,* or *SSRIs.* As with the tricyclics, this effect on serotonin in the synapse seems to have effects on the receptors, and there is some evidence that serotonin is actually the more important neurotransmitter in the treatment of depression. The development of these new agents, which help with depression but seem to work differently from the tricyclics, has provided more clues to the underlying biology of the mood disorders.

TABLE 7-2 Selective Serotonin Reuptake Inhibitors (SSRIs)

Pharmaceutical Name	Brand Name	Usual Dose (mg/day)
Fluoxetine	Prozac	20–40
Fluvoxamine	Luvox	100–200
Paroxetine	Paxil	20–60
Sertraline	Zoloft	100–150
Venlafaxine	Effexor	75–225

Note: Side effects can include nausea, overstimulation, and sexual dysfunction.

The main side effect of these medications is gastrointestinal discomfort. Many patients experience nausea for the first couple of days after starting one of the SSRIs, and a few have diarrhea or vomiting. Fortunately these side effects tend to pass quickly. These medications, especially fluoxetine, are also somewhat stimulating in some people, and while this is just what is needed by some depressed patients, others feel unpleasantly nervous or "wired" on these medications. The converse can also be seen, and sleepiness can sometimes be a side effect. Many patients report that SSRIs seem to curb their appetite a bit and notice some weight loss, especially early on in taking an SSRI. All of these side effects are usually noticed by patients pretty much immediately if they are going to occur at all, and none of them sneaks up after a person has been on an SSRI for weeks or months.

One problem, though, that might not be noticeable to patients until they've been on an SSRI for weeks or months is a change in sexual functioning, specifically a noticeable decrease in sexual interest (loss of libido) or difficulty in reaching orgasm. The frequency of these problems is difficult to gauge, because these sorts of side effects were often not asked about during clinical trials with these medications. But as more patients have been treated with SSRIs during the last decade, it has become apparent that this is a significant problem affecting about one-third of patients. There are a variety of strategies for dealing with these problems when they occur, so they should be reported to the physician. Weekend "vacations" from the medication have been reported to be helpful, as well as the addition of other medications that seem to block these effects, but sometimes a switch to another antidepressant in another class is the only solution.

When I asked one of my male patients if he was having any sexual dysfunction from his new antidepressant, he replied that he thought fluoxetine had *improved* his sex life, increasing his sexual stamina and causing him to have more intense orgasms—a reminder that a list of potential side effects should never be a reason not to try a particular medication. Pleasant sur-

TABLE 7-3 More New Antidepressants

Pharmaceutical Name	Brand Name	Usual Dose (mg/day)
Bupropion	Wellbutrin	200–300
Nefazodone	Serzone	200–400
Mirtazapine	Remeron	15–30

prises sometimes do occur. Moreover, a medication effect that causes problems for some patients can actually be helpful for others; for example, SSRIs have been reported to be helpful in treating premature ejaculation.[1]

Other New Antidepressants

Since the early 1990s a whole series of new antidepressants have come on the market that aren't tricyclics and aren't SSRIs. Since most of these pharmaceuticals don't really share many common features, there isn't a very good class name for them, although you'll sometimes see many of them listed as "atypical" or "second-generation" antidepressants. They have a variety of effects on norepinephrine, serotonin, and even other neurotransmitters; some have more than one effect on these systems, and so they are thought to provide different ways of manipulating the chemical systems in the brain concerned with mood. Their side-effect profiles vary widely as well, some having a profile more like tricyclics, others a profile more like SSRIs.

Monoamine Oxidase Inhibitors (MAOIs)

In the early 1950s a new drug that had been developed for the treatment of tuberculosis was observed to cause mood elevation in some patients who took it for their lung disease. After several more years of investigations, mostly in England, several papers appeared that confirmed the therapeutic effects of iproniazid in patients suffering from depression. Shortly afterward it was discovered that iproniazid caused inactivation of an enzyme in the body that metabolized amine compounds in the nervous system. This enzyme, called *monoamine oxidase,* is responsible for gobbling up molecules of norepinephrine, serotonin, and several other neurotransmitters. Inactivating monoamine oxidase has the effect of increasing the amounts of these compounds in the nervous system, and this effect, in some as yet poorly understood way, may be the mechanism by which such pharmaceuticals alleviate the symptoms of depression. This effect on the enzyme gives this class of pharmaceuticals their name: *monoamine oxidase inhibitors,* or *MAOIs.*

TABLE 7-4 Monoamine Oxidase Inhibitors (MAOIs)

Pharmaceutical Name	Brand Name	Usual Dose (mg/day)
Phenelzine	Nardil	30–60
Tranylcypromine	Parnate	20–30
Selegiline	Eldepryl	10

Note: Side effects can include insomnia, excess perspiration, overstimulation, lightheadedness, weight gain, water retention, and sexual dysfunction. Special diet required.

Monoamine oxidase is also present in the lining of the intestine and in the liver because a number of naturally occurring substances in various foods are close enough chemically to norepinephrine to need deactivation before they are absorbed into the bloodstream. The importance of this becomes clear when you consider that another name for norepinephrine is *adrenaline.* Tyramine, an amino acid that has adrenaline-like effects on blood pressure and heart rate, is present in high enough concentrations in some foods to cause dangerous cardiovascular problems in persons on MAOIs. A number of pharmaceuticals, including the ingredients of many over-the-counter remedies, also have adrenaline-like effects. People taking MAOIs therefore need to observe certain dietary restrictions and, even more important, *scrupulously* read the labels of any over-the-counter medication they are considering—or better yet, consult their pharmacist before taking any pharmaceutical they buy over the counter. MAOIs also interact with other medications that are prescribed or commonly used in emergency rooms for various problems. People taking MAOIs must be sure to inform all their treating physicians of this fact and should consider wearing an alerting bracelet that can communicate to ER personnel, should they be brought unconscious into an emergency room after an accident or sudden illness, that they are taking an MAOI.

MAOIs have other side effects, too. They can be stimulating and cause nervousness, insomnia, and excess perspiration. Dizzy spells, especially when suddenly getting up from lying down, can occur. MAOIs block a blood-pressure reflex that usually maintains blood pressure when we stand up, and the sudden drop in blood pressure upon standing (called orthostatic hypotension) causes lightheadedness. Weight gain, water retention, and sexual dysfunction occur as well.

As the foregoing might predict, MAOIs are seldom used in the United States unless other antidepressants have failed to be effective. Nevertheless, they are sometimes uniquely effective. I think every psychiatrist I've ever spoken with has had the experience of effectively treating a particular patient with an MAOI after no other antidepressant had helped.

TABLE 7-5 Foods to Avoid While Taking MAOIs

Alcoholic drinks, especially beer and wine
Alcohol-free beer
Fava or broad beans
Aged cheese (cream and cottage cheeses permitted)
Beef or chicken liver
Orange pulp
Pickled or smoked fish, poultry, or meats
Sauerkraut
Packaged soups
Fermented bean curd (tofu)
Yeast and protein dietary supplements
Meat extracts (e.g. Marmite, Bovril)
Summer (dry) sausage (e.g. pepperoni)
Soy sauce
Sour cream
Bananas
Avocados
Eggplant
Plums
Raisins
Spinach
Tomatoes
Yogurt

Note: This list is not exhaustive, and some items on it are low enough in tyramine that some physicians allow one or two servings per day. Get a complete list and discuss the specifics of the diet with a knowledgeable physician and pharmacist before you start on an MAOI.

Treating Bipolar Depression

The observation that antidepressants can cause manic symptoms in persons with bipolar disorder has been confirmed again and again. Perhaps more worrisome is the observation that antidepressants can cause an acceleration of the illness in some patients. Some persons with bipolar disorder experience increased cycling of their mood episodes and can even switch into a period of rapid cycling. On the other hand, antidepressants can be safely taken for symptoms of bipolar depression by many patients. When a bipolar patient becomes depressed, how does the psychiatrist decide whether or not to prescribe an antidepressant?

Studies on the issue of precipitation of mania and rapid cycling indicate that some patients are more at risk than others for a worsening of their situation with antidepressant treatment. Unfortunately it is not possible to say with certainty who is and who is not at risk. Bipolar I patients seem to be at greater risk than bipolar II patients; women are at greater risk than men; and patients who already have a history of more rapid cycling—either more full-blown episodes, or a tendency toward cyclothymia (continuous low-amplitude cycling) between full-blown episodes—are at greater risk than other patients.[2] Moreover, some antidepressant medications seem to be riskier than others. A few studies indicate that bupropion, paroxetine, and MAOIs may be safer than other antidepressants, that is, less likely to precipitate mania (and, by implication, perhaps less likely to increase cycling).[3]

In chapters 10 and 11 I discuss two treatments for depression that do not have these risks. These are electroconvulsive therapy (ECT) and psychotherapy. These treatments are often avoided or overlooked in the treatment of bipolar depression, ECT often thought of as "too drastic," and psychotherapy dismissed because "talking can't help." As I hope to convince you, neither of these attitudes is justified by the research.

Perhaps more than any other treatment issue, the questions surrounding the use of antidepressants in bipolar disorder emphasize the need for individualization of treatment for every patient. There are no hard-and-fast rules for when, why, or how to use antidepressant medications in bipolar patients. Patient and physician need to communicate clearly and honestly about every aspect of symptoms and treatment in order to achieve the best treatment outcome.

CHAPTER 8

Antipsychotic Medications

A DIFFICULTY THAT IMMEDIATELY ARISES IN DISCUSSING THE ANTI-psychotic medications is their unfortunate name. *Psychotic* is an imprecise term at best, and these medications have many more uses than simply treating psychotic symptoms.

When I was training at Johns Hopkins, all the residents knew better than to describe a patient as "psychotic" within earshot of Hopkins' chairman of psychiatry, Paul McHugh. "What does *that* word mean? You might as well call the patient 'crazy!'" I can hear him say. "What are you trying to say: Is the patient delusional? Hallucinated? Disoriented? Does he have a disorder of thinking? *What?*" Dr. McHugh's point is that we have very good words to describe the various symptoms of major mental illnesses, and that to describe a person as suffering from "psychosis" simply doesn't say very much. Nevertheless, *psychosis* is such a frequently used word in works on psychiatric disorders that we need to agree on some sort of definition in order to understand what is usually meant by it.

A psychosis can be thought of as a mental state or disorder in which the affected person's ability to comprehend his or her environment and react to it appropriately is severely impaired. The layman's definition of *psychotic* might be "out of touch with reality." The person who is hearing voices (hallucinating) or who has bizarre idiosyncratic beliefs (delusions) is psychotic. The word also connotes a severe disorganization of thinking and behavior, usually with restlessness and agitation. The manic syndrome is a good example of a state of psychosis, and we have already talked about "psychotic features" in depression.

In the 1930s a group of pharmaceutical compounds called *phenothiazines* were synthesized in Europe and were found to have antihistamine and sedative properties. One in particular, chlorpromazine, was found to be very useful in surgical anaesthesia because it deepened anaesthetic sedation more safely than other available agents. In the early 1950s two French psychiatrists carried out several clinical trials using chlorpromazine to treat highly agitated patients suffering from schizophrenia and mania. They had hoped that the drug would provide sedation for these very sick patients, which it did—but these astute clinicians noticed that this medication did much more.

In addition to its quieting and sleep-promoting effects, chlorpromazine made the hallucinations and bizarre delusional beliefs of many patients with schizophrenia practically disappear. It also decreased the severity of the disorganization of thinking and the agitated behavior seen in patients with acute mania. Chlorpromazine, in other words, had a *specific* effect on the cluster of symptoms usually referred to as "psychotic" symptoms, and thus the name for this group came about: *antipsychotic medications*. Occasionally they are still referred to as *neuroleptic* medications (or *neuroleptics*), from *neuroleptique*, the French word coined from Greek roots that means roughly "affecting the nervous system." The term *major tranquilizers* was frequently used for these medications at one time—with the term *minor tranquilizers* used for sleep and anxiety medications—but these agents are much more than just "tranquilizers," and this term has fortunately fallen out of favor. As we shall see, their effects are more than simply "antipsychotic," but until a better term comes along, *antipsychotic medications* is what we're stuck with.

Therapeutic Profile

Episodes of bipolar disorder—both depression and mania—can sometimes include extremely frightening mental symptoms and dangerously disturbed behaviors. But as we saw in chapters 6 and 7, mood stabilizers and antidepressants sometimes take weeks to begin working. What can be done to slow down the racing thoughts, the pressured, bursting overactivity of the manic patient before lithium starts working? What can be done to help the psychotically depressed patient tormented by hallucinations before the antidepressant starts working? This is where antipsychotic medications come in. Because their calming effects begin almost *immediately,* these medications are especially useful in acute mania and are frequently part of the treatment for the severely ill manic patient. In cases of depression wherein the patient is highly restless and agitated, they can have similar beneficial effects.

The controversy with these medications is whether they have more than a nonspecific calming effect on patients—whether they have an antipsychotic effect above and beyond their effects as tranquilizers. There is some evidence that high doses of the less powerful medications used to treat anxiety disorders might be just as useful to treat acute and severe symptoms.[1] Nevertheless, because these medications are very effective and usually used for only a short time, they remain an important adjunct treatment for many patients with severe symptomatology.

The main chemical effect of all of the pharmaceuticals in this class is a blocking of dopamine receptors in the brain. Neural circuits that use dopamine as their neurotransmitter may be dysfunctional in some way in people with schizophrenia, causing the bizarre hallucinations and disorders of thinking typical of that illness, and these medications may work by affecting these systems in some as yet unknown way. Whether or not these medications alleviate in a similar fashion the psychotic symptoms that sometimes complicate bipolar disorder is as yet unknown.

After the development of the original group of antipsychotic medications, the phenothiazines, several other potent dopamine-blocking medications were developed in the 1960s and 1970s. The side-effect profile of these newer medications was marginally better than that of the phenothiazines, but they did not represent much of an advance therapeutically.

More recently, however, several new antipsychotic medications have been introduced that not only have a substantially better side-effect profile but also seem to represent a substantial therapeutic advance over older agents. We'll discuss these in a bit, but first I want to review the side-effect profile of the more traditionally used antipsychotic medications.

TABLE 8-1 Traditional Antipsychotic Medications

Pharmaceutical Name	Brand Name
Chlorpromazine	Thorazine
Fluphenazine	Prolixen
Haloperidol	Haldol
Loxapine	Loxitane
Molindone	Moban
Perphenazine	Trilafon
Thioridazine	Mellaril
Thiothixene	Navane
Trifluoperazine	Stelazine

Note: Side effects include sedation, anticholinergic effects, and extrapyramidal effects (see text).
    This table does not include "usual doses" because these medications are usually used for brief periods of time and often on an "as-needed" basis in the treatment of mood disorders. Doses are individualized to the needs of each patient and vary widely.

Side Effects

The original antipsychotic medications were called "major tranquilizers" at one time because they are—well, tranquilizers, in a major way. Some are more sedating than others, but all can be pretty powerful sedatives, especially in higher doses. They can cause some of the same anticholinergic side effects as tricyclic antidepressants: dry mouth, constipation, blurred vision. People seem to accommodate to these side effects after a period that ranges from days to weeks.

The main problem with most of these medications is their effect on muscle tone and movement, side effects that are caused by the dopamine blockade these agents cause. In textbook discussions of these medications you will see these problems referred to as *extrapyramidal symptoms,* or simply *EPS.* Dopamine is the main neurotransmitter used in a complex circuit of brain areas called the *extrapyramidal system,* which coordinates movement. The name contrasts this system with another brain system that is called the *pyramidal system* because its main fibers are carried in triangular-shaped bundles into the spinal cord (the "spinal pyramids" or "pyramidal tract"). The pyramidal system controls the quick, accurate execution of fine muscle movement, and the extrapyramidal system makes sure that the rest of the body moves as needed for the smooth and graceful execution of these movements. Antipsychotic medications, by blocking the dopamine receptors in these centers, cause several movement problems. One is *pseudo-parkinsonism.* In Parkinson's disease there is a degeneration of part of the extrapyramidal system: the death of dopamine neurons in one of its crucial components, a brain area called the *substantia nigra.* You may know that persons suffering from Parkinson's disease have a slowed and shuffling walk, seem to lose facial expression because of stiffness in their face muscles, and also have trembling of their hands. Pseudo-parkinsonism consists of these same symptoms. The neurons don't die as they do in the disease, but their chemical messenger, dopamine, is blocked from doing its work by a pharmaceutical agent.

Another set of extrapyramidal side effects are *acute dystonic reactions.* These are muscular spasms that usually involve the tongue and facial and neck muscles, and they are more common in young male patients than in others. People taking antipsychotic medications can also develop a very uncomfortable restlessness called *akathesia.* This is felt mostly in the legs, and the individual feels the need to walk or pace.

Fortunately these side effects are all treatable, either by lowering the dose of medication or by adding one of several medications that are also used to treat Parkinson's disease. Although uncomfortable, they are not dangerous, and they usually respond quickly to treatment once they are encountered and identified.

Most of these medications can, over years, cause a side effect called *tardive dyskinesia,* or *TD* for short. This consists of repetitive involuntary movements, usually of the facial muscles—usually chewing, blinking, or lip-pursing movements. There is no good treatment for TD other than discontinuing the medication. We used to worry a lot about TD, because some patients who developed it seemed to continue to have these movements even after the medication was stopped. But two factors are calming these worries: the discovery that most TD symptoms *do* eventually go away with time and, more important, the development of new antipsychotic medications that do not seem to cause TD. We'll talk about them in the next section of this chapter.

I want to emphasize that extrapyramidal symptoms sound a lot worse than they are, are usually easily treated, and are not dangerous. On the other hand, the symptoms of bipolar disorder that antipsychotic medications are typically used to treat *are* extremely dangerous and much more uncomfortable. These medications are powerful agents, and they need to be used carefully and for the shortest period of time possible, but for the present, at least, they are nearly irreplaceable in treating the most dangerous and most terrible symptoms of severe mania and psychotic depression.

The New Antipsychotic Medications

It's probably apparent to you after reading the foregoing paragraphs that there's room for improvement in the antipsychotic medications. Not only are the extrapyramidal symptoms uncomfortable until treated, but it is usually necessary to add another medication to control them—and the more different medications a person takes, the more likely he or she is to have problems with side effects and drug interactions. So it created quite a stir when a new group of antipsychotic medications was introduced which doesn't seem to cause EPS. Even more good news: they seem to work better than their predecessors. One article in the *American Journal of Psychiatry* called the first of these new agents "arguably the most significant development in antipsychotic drug therapy since the advent of chlorpromazine."[2]

These agents are called *atypical antipsychotic medications* because although they block dopamine receptors just as their predecessors do (though not as potently), they differ from the typical antipsychotic medications in that they are also active at serotonin receptors. This seems to have two effects: extrapyramidal symptoms do not appear nearly as often, and these medications seem to have significant mood-stabilizing effects.

The first atypical antipsychotic, clozapine, was synthesized in the laboratory in the 1960s but was not marketed in the United States until 1990. One of the reasons it took so long for clozapine to get onto the market is that it causes a very dangerous drop in the number of white blood cells (called *agranulo-*

TABLE 8-2 New Antipsychotic Medications

Pharmaceutical Name	Brand Name
Clozapine	Clozaril
Olanzapine	Zyprexa
Quetiapine	Seroquel
Risperidone	Risperdal
Ziprasidone	Zeldox

Note: This table does not include "usual doses" because these medications are usually used for brief periods of time and often on an "as-needed" basis in the treatment of mood disorders. Doses are individualized to the needs of each patient and vary widely.

cytosis) in about 1 percent of the patients who take it.[3] This problem might have meant the end of the line for clozapine were it not for the fact that it was found to be highly effective in treating patients with schizophrenia who derived no benefit from traditional antipsychotic medications. Dramatic case studies of patients with chronic treatment-resistant schizophrenia basically "awakening" from years of unrelenting psychotic symptoms after they started clozapine sustained the interest of clinicians and pharmaceutical researchers. When it was discovered that the risk of agranulocytosis could be substantially reduced if the patient had his or her white blood cell count monitored on a weekly basis, clozapine treatment became more available to larger groups of patients, and it was not long before treatment-resistant mood-disorder patients were being treated with it as well.

There are now several studies of the use of clozapine in people with treatment-resistant bipolar and schizoaffective disorder. A year after clozapine came onto the market, a letter to the editor of the *Journal of Clinical Psychopharmacology* reported that clozapine had been effective in treating two rapid-cycling bipolar patients "who were resistant to all conventional treatment."[4] One patient was a forty-eight-year-old woman who had been very ill for more than thirty years, had started rapid cycling about five years previously, and had been almost constantly cycling between delusional depressions and dysphoric mania for a whole year before starting on clozapine. The authors stated that after the woman had been taking clozapine alone for three months, "her mood swings completely stopped." The case report indicates that there were episodes of breakthrough manic and depressive symptoms, but the patient had done remarkably better on clozapine. (This case illustrates why, for some patients at least, weekly blood tests are a price worth paying.)

Another study looked at twenty-five acutely manic patients "for whom lithium, anticonvulsants and [traditional] neuroleptics had been ineffective, had produced intolerable side effects, or both."[5] Almost three-quarters of these patients had "marked improvement" in their manic symptoms. Clozapine was even more effective in the bipolar patients without rapid cycling than in the rapid cyclers and the schizoaffective patients. The answer to the question posed in a 1995 article titled "Is Clozapine a Mood Stabilizer?"[6] seems to be an emphatic yes. A number of studies have indicated that clozapine has unique benefits in the treatment of bipolar disorder.

In the years following the introduction of clozapine, other atypical antipsychotic medications have come along. None of them causes the blood count problem that clozapine does, and so weekly blood tests are not necessary with these medications. It remains to be seen whether or not these new agents are as helpful as clozapine for bipolar-disorder patients, but there are hopeful signs.

Of the other atypical antipsychotic medications listed in table 8-2, olanzapine is the most similar to clozapine in its effects on different neurotransmitter systems, leading some researchers to consider it especially promising. It has already been shown to have some mood-stabilizing effects in patients diagnosed with schizoaffective disorder.[7]

Although they do not seem to cause EPS, the newer antipsychotic medications can cause the other side effects that the traditional antipsychotic medications cause: anticholinergic side effects and sedation.

After many years of "nothing new" as far as antipsychotic agents are concerned, many new drugs are in development. Better antipsychotic medications are surely among them, and hope remains high that more will be found to be of special benefit in the treatment of bipolar disorder.

CHAPTER 9

Other Medications, Hormones, and an Herb

A NUMBER OF OTHER PHARMACEUTICAL AGENTS HAVE ATTRACTED AT-tention because they have been proven helpful in the treatment of bipolar symptoms. Others seem to show promise—or have promised more than they have delivered—and warrant a discussion as well.

Benzodiazepine Medications

The benzodiazepine medications represented a major advance in the treatment of psychiatric symptoms when they were first developed, and they continue to be widely prescribed. They often have a place in the treatment of bipolar disorder because they are highly effective for the treatment of anxiety and insomnia and, in higher doses, are safe and effective sedatives. If this sounds too good to be true and you're wondering if there's a hidden drawback, there is. These medications can be abused, and it's possible to become psychologically dependent on and even physically addicted to them. (Withdrawal symptoms in persons taking high doses of these medications can include very serious problems like seizures.) Moreover, their sedating effects decrease over time, and after several weeks of use their effectiveness as tranquilizers decreases. For these reasons benzodiazepines are best thought of as temporary measures.

Benzodiazepines really have two main uses in treating bipolar disorder: in treating patients who are very sick and in treating patients who are doing very well. This seems to be a contradiction, doesn't it? The explanation is in

TABLE 9-1 Benzodiazepine Medications

Pharmaceutical Name	Brand Name	Usual Dose (mg/day)*
Alprazolam	Xanax	0.75–1.5
Chlordiazepoxide	Librium	15–40
Clonazepam	Klonapin	1.5–3
Clorazepate	Tranxene	15–30
Diazepam	Valium	4–20
Lorazepam	Ativan	2–6

*These medications are best thought of as temporary agents and are frequently prescribed for occasional "as-needed" use. Doses are often 50 percent below these ranges or even lower.

the doses used and how these medications are combined with other medications. In acutely manic patients, the short-acting benzodiazepine lorazepam (Ativan) can be an effective short-term tranquilizer, especially in combination with a traditional antipsychotic medication like haloperidol (Haldol). This combination is very familiar to psychiatrists working in emergency settings because it works quickly and effectively in calming even the most agitated patients. A very ill manic patient, perhaps delusional and agitated, who hasn't slept for days can be asleep less than an hour after receiving this combination, especially in injectable form. The longer-acting benzodiazepine clonazepam (Klonapin) has also been used and extensively studied in the treatment of acute manic symptoms and appears also to be an effective adjunct medication.

These medications are not mood stabilizers and are not effective in treating hallucinations or delusions, but as sedatives they are unsurpassed. Remember that before effective psychiatric medications became available, patients with severe mania died of the physical stress of the manic state. By simply slowing manic patients down for a few hours or days until antipsychotic medications and mood-stabilizing medications start working, benzodiazepines can be literally lifesaving.

At the other end of the spectrum of illness severity, patients who are not having severe mood symptoms can safely take these medications for anxiety symptoms and insomnia. As we shall see in part IV of this book, anxiety and psychological stress can make bipolar patients more susceptible to an episode of their mood disorder (as can sleep deprivation). During periods of unavoidable psychological stress, such as after the death of a loved one, benzodiazepine medications can help with the insomnia and lessen the psychological tension that can bring on mood symptoms in bipolar patients. It's important to emphasize here that these medications should not be used as substitutes for making changes to chronically stressful situations. A person who finds that he or she needs a sedative to deal with usual everyday situations is well on his or her way to psychological dependence on tranquilizers, medication abuse, and addiction. We'll discuss this in more depth in chapter 15.

There's another way these medications are used, and that is in treating patients who have anxiety disorders. Anxiety disorders (such as recurrent panic attacks) are effectively treated with benzodiazepines. The connections between the mood disorders and anxiety disorders are poorly understood, but there are certainly some people who need treatment for both. The treatment of panic disorder and other severe anxiety disorders sometimes involves taking benzodiazepine medications on a more long-term basis, but prolonged use of benzodiazepines is the exception rather than the rule in treating bipolar disorders, and any use requires close monitoring.

Calcium-Channel-Blocking Agents

Since the 1970s, scientists researching bipolar disorder have been interested in a group of medications called calcium channel blockers. The flow of calcium ions is instrumental in the electrical activity of cells, and these medications modulate this flow by blockading the channels through which the calcium ions move into the cell. These medications are widely used in the treatment of heart problems. Like nerve cells, muscle cells are active electrically, and calcium channel blockers have powerful effects on the tiny muscle cells that open and close blood vessels. Blocking the calcium channels of these cells has the effect of relaxing them, allowing the arteries to open more and blood flow through them to increase. This is a very useful effect in treating coronary artery disease and angina—chest pains caused by too little flow through the coronary arteries, the arteries that supply the heart—as well as in treating high blood pressure, heart failure, and abnormal heart rhythms. The most widely prescribed calcium-channel-blocking agents are verapamil (Calan, Isoptin, and Verelan), nimodipine (Nimotop), nifedipine (Adalac and Procardia), diltiazem (Cardizem), and amlodipine (Norvasc).

These agents can be thought of as having a calming effect on electrical cells, analogous in some ways to the effect of anticonvulsants. So it didn't take long for clinical researchers to look into the effects of calcium-blocking agents on mania. A case report appeared in 1982 describing a therapeutic effect of verapamil in treating a manic patient.[1] Since then, several more reports and series of controlled trials in several hundreds of patients have appeared.[2] These reports suggest that some of the calcium channel blockers may be effective antimanic agents for some patients, but the superiority of these agents over lithium remains unproven. Many of the studies were of only several weeks' duration, so the mood-stabilizing effects of these agents over time remain largely unknown as well. There is practically no research on the antidepressant effects of these medications.

Psychiatrists have not rushed to use calcium channel blockers on bipolar patients, possibly because there is so much more research on lithium and other agents. Since calcium channel blockers don't appear to offer any special advantages over the medications we are more familiar with and that have a longer track record, there has been little impetus to do more research on them.

Might calcium channel blockers have a place in the treatment of patients who have bipolar disorder and who also have heart or blood-pressure problems? Will one agent effectively treat both conditions in some people? The problem here is that psychiatrists aren't usually very experienced in managing heart disease, and cardiologists aren't very experienced in managing bipolar disorder, so if we attempt to manage both problems with one medication, the treatment of one or the other will suffer. Moreover, both bipolar disorder and most heart and blood-pressure disorders are long-term conditions that often require a shift in treatment approaches over time, and this can cause any number of problems. For example, if a hypertensive bipolar patient's verapamil needs to be switched to another type of blood-pressure medication because it isn't working anymore, the last thing he or she needs is to risk a manic episode by going off the mood-stabilizing medication. Should the patient be put on a new antihypertensive and a new mood stabilizer simultaneously? If side effects appear, which medication is to blame?

I include this section on the calcium-channel-blocking agents simply because most books and papers on the treatment of bipolar disorders mention them and cite a report or two on their use in some unusual group of patients.[3] But at this point, routine use of these agents is not usually recommended.[4]

Stimulant Medications

For many years the treatment of depression often included the use of powerful medications known as psychostimulants. Amphetamine, the prototype compound, is perhaps the best known of this group. These medications boost energy levels, concentration, and mood, and a number of years ago they were frequently prescribed for patients with depression. As psychiatrists became more sophisticated in using antidepressants, and as more antidepressants became available in the 1970s—and perhaps more significantly, when the many problems with amphetamine-like drugs become more apparent—their use in the treatment of mood disorders fell out of favor.

The problems with these medications are their tendency to raise blood pressure and their abuse potential. Because they increase wakefulness and improve concentration and physical endurance, they were widely abused by long-distance drivers, athletes, college students cramming for exams, and other persons trying to improve their performance at any cost. Amphetamines tend to lose their stimulating effects with prolonged use, can cause symptoms of paranoia indistinguishable from paranoid schizophrenia, and when stopped after prolonged use or use of high doses frequently cause the abuser to crash into a severe, even suicidal depression.

As with a number of powerful and highly effective treatments for psychiatric symptoms, enthusiastic overuse led to abuse and discredit for these medications, which in turn led to underutilization of an effective treatment and even denial of it to patients who could benefit from it; physicians were reluctant to prescribe what had come to be seen as a "bad" pharmaceutical. But as usually happens with enough time and enough good research, the pendulum has swung back toward the center, and the legitimate and safe uses of psychostimulants have become established. (A similar chain of events unfolded for electroconvulsive therapy, as we'll see in the next chapter.)

The use of psychostimulants as adjuncts to other treatments has become established in the approach to treatment-resistant depression, depression in the elderly, and also depression associated with medical illnesses such as cancer and AIDS.[5] Their use in bipolar depression is not as well defined, but cautious use in bipolar patients with treatment-resistant depression has been recommended.[6] There have been reports of mania induced by stimulants, warranting special caution in patients with frequent or severe manic episodes.[7] Psychostimulants are safe when used as prescribed, although side effects can include headache, flushing, loss of appetite, and insomnia. The severe problems noted in the preceding paragraphs are usually associated with prolonged use of high doses.

Another interesting use of psychostimulants has recently been reported: as treatment for the sexual dysfunction caused by SSRI antidepressant medications.[8] One small study found dextroamphetamine or methylphenidate to be 80 percent effective in reversing the sexual dysfunction caused by a serotonin reuptake inhibitor in twenty-four patients. (It should be mentioned here that psychostimulants are not the only remedy for sexual dysfunction symptoms caused by SSRIs; see chapter 7.)

TABLE 9-2 Psychostimulant Medications

Pharmaceutical Name	Brand Name	Usual Dose (mg/day)
Dextroamphetamine	Dexedrine	10–20
Methylphenidate	Ritalin	20–30
Pemoline	Cylert	56.25–75

Note: Side effects include headache, flushing, loss of appetite, and insomnia.

Thyroid Hormones

In several sections of this book we're going to talk about the interrelationships of mood and hormones. The pulsing daily rhythms of melatonin from the pineal gland that may be involved with the seasonal mood changes of seasonal affective disorder (SAD), the mood fluctuations that can follow changing levels of female reproductive hormones (important in understanding postpartum mood symptoms and premenstrual syndromes), the stress hormones secreted by the adrenal gland—all these hormones appear to be important in the regulation of mood. But perhaps the most important in this respect are the thyroid hormones.

The thyroid gland plays a major role in the body's energy regulation. Too little thyroid gland activity leads to sluggishness and weight gain and too much to metabolic overdrive—rapid pulse, nervous energy, and anxiety. While the precise role of thyroid hormones in the regulation of mood remains unclear, it's very clear that normal thyroid functioning is essential for effective treatment of mood disorders. Put another way, if a patient's mood symptoms don't respond to the usual treatments, or if a treatment that has been effective seems to lose its effectiveness, a thyroid problem, especially abnormally low thyroid functioning (hypothyroidism), should be suspected.

Several studies have shown that hypothyroidism is surprisingly common in patients with rapid-cycling bipolar disorder.[9] One group of scientists tested for thyroid abnormalities using stored blood samples from almost four thousand patients who had been hospitalized for psychiatric problems over a period of four years. They found a high association between thyroid abnormalities and a diagnosis of rapid-cycling bipolar disorder.[10] But it is also clear that some rapid-cycling bipolar patients whose thyroid hormone levels prove to be in the "normal" range when blood tests are done can nevertheless benefit from treatment with thyroid medications. It is thought that thyroid medication somehow makes these patients more responsive to other treatments. Patients who have a partial response to lithium or other mood stabilizers may have better control of their mood symptoms when thyroid medication is added, even if their thyroid hormones levels are normal. As a paper on treating rapid-cycling bipolar disorder put it, "Normal thyroid [blood test results] should not discourage the clinician from pursuing thyroid supplementation" in rapid-cycling bipolar patients.[11]

At one time it was thought that very high doses of thyroid medication—enough to make the patient slightly hyperthyroid—were necessary to obtain this effect, but this approach now seems unnecessarily risky. Patients seem to benefit just as much from usual doses. For more on thyroid hormones and mood disorders, see "Mood Disorders due to Hormonal Problems" in chapter 18.

St. John's Wort

Some of our most important pharmaceuticals are synthetic duplications of naturally occurring compounds—often, compounds originally discovered in medicinal plants. Many of these compounds had been used therapeutically as herbal preparations for centuries before modern chemical methods became available to identify the plant's active ingredients and allow synthetic mass production. Aspirin is purified salicylic acid, found in the bark of willow trees; the heart medication digitalis originally came from the garden foxglove plant, *Digitalis purpurea;* the antimalarial agent quinine and the heart medication quinidine are found in the bark of the cinchona tree; the list goes on and on.

Yet another plant extract seems poised to become the basis for new medications in the near future, this time for a psychiatric condition. There is growing interest in the antidepressant properties of preparations of *Hypericum perforatum,* commonly known as St. John's wort, one of about three hundred *Hypericum* species: shrubby perennial plants with bright yellow flowers that grow in most temperate regions of the world.

Teas and other extracts of St. John's wort have been recommended by herbalists for centuries to treat everything from insomnia to the painful viral skin infection called shingles. In the late 1980s hypericum was investigated as a possible treatment for HIV infection when it was discovered that it had activity against retroviruses, activity that unfortunately did not translate into clinical usefulness against HIV infection. The results of clinical investigations of hypericum's antidepressant efficacy, however, are much more promising.

Most of the scientific work so far on hypericum has been done in Germany, where herbal preparations are more widely available and, perhaps, are more seriously regarded as valid treatment options for serious illnesses. Several studies have been done comparing hypericum extracts with a placebo and with a standard antidepressant. The results of these studies are generally quite encouraging and indicate that hypericum extracts have an antidepressant effect that is clinically significant in some people. A 1996 article in the *British Medical Journal* systematically reviewed twenty-three different studies involving a total of 1,757 patients and concluded that "extracts of hypericum are more effective than placebo for the treatment of mild to moderately severe depressive disorders."[12] This paper indicated that patients taking hypericum preparations generally reported fewer and less severe side effects than those taking standard antidepressants.

Much work remains to be done to determine which groups of patients will benefit from hypericum and which patients should be treated with better-established agents. Problems with the design of many of the available studies make it difficult to compare the effectiveness of hypericum and pharmaceutical antidepressants. For example, in two studies comparing hypericum with the tricyclic antidepressants imipramine and amitriptyline in patients with depression, the prescribed doses of the antidepressants in the studies were low—so low, in fact, that they would be considered ineffective by most psychiatrists.[13] Another problem is that these studies often lump together patients with mild depression and patients with more severe depression, making it difficult to know what kinds of depression hypericum is helpful for: mildly depressed patients, more severely depressed patients, or both. Perhaps most important, there are no studies looking at the use of hypericum in bipolar depression—at least not as of this writing.

At present it is difficult to recommend hypericum preparations for persons with bipolar disorder. There are simply not enough rigorously controlled studies of its therapeutic effects in persons with major mood disorders—and as we have seen, antidepressants are not without risk in bipolar disorder. People who suffer from mild unipolar depression symptoms might prudently attempt treatment of their symptoms with hypericum preparations under the supervision of a physician; those with bipolar disorder, however, are well advised to hold off on using hypericum until more information about its use in bipolar disorder becomes available.

The fact that a pharmaceutically active chemical comes from an herbal preparation does not necessarily make it safer than or superior to a chemically synthesized compound. Remember that nicotine and strychnine are found in plants, and that some of the deadliest poisons known to man, the amatoxins, occur naturally in the "deathcap" mushroom, *Amanita phalloides.*[14] The lower incidence of side effects of herbal preparations can often be attributed to the fact the active compounds are usually present in low concentrations in herbal preparations, an advantage that can be easily duplicated by using low doses of a synthetic pharmaceutical.

Nevertheless, discovery of a pharmacologically active plant compound has often formed the basis for development of a much larger number of useful new drugs and led to other exciting discoveries. The chemical isolation of opium from the poppy plant led to the development of literally dozens of safer and more potent pain medications, and also to the discovery of similar compounds in the brain (called endorphins)—forming the basis for practically an entire new branch of neurochemistry. As we learn more about hypericum, it may turn out that a whole new class of safer and more effective antidepressants will emerge derived from compounds from a plant with a pretty yellow flower growing on hillsides and in meadows all over the world.

CHAPTER 10

Electroconvulsive Therapy

ELECTROCONVULSIVE THERAPY (ECT) IS A HIGHLY EFFECTIVE TREAT-
ment for both phases of bipolar disorder, often providing dramatic and rapid
relief of symptoms even when other treatments have failed. Unfortunately
ECT is also often thought of as a "last resort" by physicians, and patients and
their families resist its use because of myths and misconceptions about it.

Too often the popular media refer to ECT as "shock treatments," with all
the unpleasant connotations of that term: *shock* defined as an unpleasant jolt
or blow, or reminding you of the painful spark of static electricity that comes
from touching a doorknob after crossing a carpeted room on a dry winter day.
Calling ECT "shock treatments" is a bit like referring to modern surgery as
"knife treatments"—accurate in a crude sort of way, but doing injustice to
what is now a safe and effective treatment that can be literally lifesaving. That's
not to gloss over the fact that ECT was crude and unpleasant in its early days—
though not nearly as unpleasant as surgery was in *its* early days—but modern anaesthetic techniques have changed all that.

Although the effectiveness of ECT in mood disorders was not a completely accidental discovery, its original theoretical basis has been shown to
have no validity, so the development of modern ECT was a kind of happy accident. In the early 1930s the Hungarian physician Joseph Ladislas von
Meduna proposed that there was a mutual antagonism between epilepsy and
schizophrenia: patients who suffered from epilepsy did not suffer from schizophrenia and vice versa. Modern research has shown that this is not the case,
but von Meduna—convinced of the truth of this idea on the basis of his ex-

amination of the microscopic appearance of the brains of persons with the two conditions—conducted animal experiments attempting to find a way to produce seizure activity artificially. In 1935 he published a paper reporting a dramatic improvement in symptoms after artificially inducing seizures in several patients with schizophrenia. Von Meduna had used injections to produce seizures, but several years later two Italian psychiatrists reported that seizures could be produced by briefly passing a low-voltage electrical current through the skull by means of electrodes applied to the scalp. Ugo Cerletti and Lucio Bini had developed their technique in animals and then tried it with several patients with schizophrenia, and they also reported remarkable success.

Although patients with some forms of schizophrenia did indeed often show improvement in some of their symptoms after these treatments, it quickly became apparent that severely depressed patients showed improvement that was little short of miraculous. Decades previously Emil Kraepelin had described patients in a catatonic state from depression: "The patients lie in bed taking no interest in anything. They betray no pronounced emotion; they are mute, inaccessible; they pass their [bowel movements] under them; they stare straight in front of them with [a] vacant expression of countenance like a mask and with wide open eyes."[1] With "electroshock" treatments, such patients had complete recovery from their symptoms within a matter of days. The last major breakthrough in the treatment of psychiatric problems—the discovery of the Wassermann test for syphilis more than thirty years earlier— now seemed almost insignificant compared with this astonishing new therapeutic technique. Naturally, interest in ECT spread quickly around the globe.

But ECT's success was also its near downfall. Like many seemingly miraculous treatments, it was overprescribed at first and probably administered to many hundreds of persons it had little chance of helping. It's important to remember, however, that these were desperate times in psychiatry. With the discovery of antipsychotic medications nearly a decade off and the discovery of antidepressants nearly two, "little chance" of helping was better than no chance at all. Since, as we shall see, ECT is a highly effective treatment for mania, some institutions were inclined to use it for any and all highly agitated patients, and sometimes on merely uncooperative ones (a misuse that was dramatized—with a few inaccuracies unfortunately thrown in—in the film *One Flew over the Cuckoo's Nest*). Another negative factor was that in the first decade or so after its development, ECT had very serious complications. An epileptic seizure is a violent event: all the muscles of the body contract simultaneously for a few moments, sometimes with such force that broken bones result. Breathing stops as well, and heart rhythm irregularities occur which can be fatal.

The nearly indiscriminate overprescription of a therapy that had serious potential side effects led to a backlash against ECT. By the late 1960s and 1970s, although modern anaesthetic techniques were making ECT safer, and more careful research was being done to determine which psychiatric disorders the treatment helped with and which it did not, the damage to ECT's reputation had already been done. (*Cuckoo's Nest,* awarded the Oscar for best movie in 1975, depicted ECT as it would have been administered circa 1945, and certainly didn't help.) State hospitals drew up regulations sharply curtailing its use, and legislation was in effect briefly in California banning the procedure completely.

Fortunately the pendulum has swung back to center. ECT is now safer than most surgical procedures, side effects are minimal, and indications for its use have been clarified. A 1980 survey of 166 ECT patients reported that about half of them thought a trip to the dentist was more unpleasant than an electroconvulsive treatment.[2]

Modern ECT

The major improvements in ECT have been due to developments in anaesthetic techniques. ECT is usually done in the recovery room of the surgical suite of a hospital, the area where patients waking up from surgery are taken for observation. This makes sense when you realize that the actual ECT treatment is over in about sixty seconds, and that most of the "treatment" time is actually the ten minutes or so it takes for the patient to awaken from general anaesthesia. Some large psychiatric hospitals have their own treatment suites that are similarly equipped.

ECT is now done under general anaesthesia just as surgery is. Because each treatment lasts only a few minutes, intravenous barbiturate is used instead of the inhaled anaesthetics used in most surgery. The crucial anaesthetic advance for ECT was the introduction in the 1950s of agents called *muscle relaxants,* or more properly *neuromuscular blocking agents.* These medications, also given intravenously, temporarily paralyze the patient by blocking nervous center transmission to the muscles. This prevents the violent muscle contractions during seizures that characterized early ECT.

Immediately before the treatment, patients usually receive an injection of a medication that prevents abnormal heart rhythms (atropine or glycopyrrolate). Then an IV is started, and the patient is given the barbiturate and then the muscle relaxant. The patient is asleep and completely relaxed in less than five minutes. Electrode disks similar to those used to take cardiograms are applied to the scalp. Modern ECT equipment designed for the purpose delivers a precisely timed and measured electrical stimulus, usually of a half-second to several seconds' duration. In *bilateral* treatments, an electrode is applied over each temple. In *unilateral* treatments, wherein the object is to stimulate only half the brain, one electrode is placed in the middle of the forehead and the other at the temple. (Unilateral treatment causes less post-ECT confusion and memory problems and is now used almost exclusively. In some rare cases it doesn't work as well, and those patients must therefore receive bilateral treatments.)

The "seizure" in modern ECT is pretty much an electrical event only, with little or none of the jerking movements that usually characterize seizures. Most ECT machines used today also record an electroencephalogram (a measurement of the electrical activity of the brain) through the same electrodes used to deliver the stimulus, so that the physician can see how long the induced "seizure" lasts—usually twenty-five to forty-five seconds. There might be a few brief muscle contractions observed during this time, but the muscle relaxant keeps the patient nearly motionless. There is usually a brief quickening of the heart rate and an increase of blood pressure that also signal that the "seizure" has occurred. The anaesthetist uses a face-mask breathing device to deliver oxygen until the patient wakes up five or ten minutes later and the treatment is over.

About the only patients who absolutely can't receive ECT are those very few individuals with medical conditions so severe that even ten to fifteen minutes of general anaesthesia is too dangerous—people with really severe cardiac or lung diseases, for example. ECT is safe in the elderly and even during pregnancy.

Patients awakening from anaesthesia are a bit groggy, of course, and many are also slightly fuzzy-headed and feel "spacey" for another hour or so. This effect is probably related to the treatments themselves, not just the anaesthesia, and it resembles the mild postseizure confusion that patients with true epilepsy sometimes experience. Occasionally a more severe period of confusion called *delirium* is seen, especially after bilateral treatments and especially toward the end of a course of treatments. Sedatives can treat this problem quickly, but when it occurs, consideration should be given to stopping the treatments or giving them less often.

The most troublesome possible side effects of ECT relate to its effect on memory: about two-thirds of patients report that ECT affects their memory in some way. The most common memory loss seen with ECT is for events occurring during the several weeks when the patient was actually receiving ECT. Since treatments are typically given three times a week and a patient typically needs six to twelve treatments for complete recovery, a course of ECT will last two to four weeks. Patients not infrequently lose memory for some events that occurred during those weeks. Patients sometimes also suffer *retrograde amnesia* as well: memory loss for a period of time before they actually started ECT. This is thought to occur because ECT somehow disrupts the process by which shorter-term memories become incorporated into longer-term memory. (If you've ever lost an hour's worth of computer work because you didn't save your work before something untoward "froze" your computer, you get the idea of what retrograde amnesia is. The short-term memories that are still in the brain's memory "buffer" are lost because of the ECT.) Patients who have successfully completed a course of ECT may report not remembering checking in to the hospital, or they might not recollect a home visit or a trip they took with their family during the treatments. This problem seems to be worst just after a patient receives ECT. In a study of forty-three patients interviewed about their memory a few weeks after completing ECT, some reported difficulty remembering events for a period up to two years before their ECT. But when these patients were tested again seven *months* after their treatment, these more distant memories had been almost completely recovered.[3]

In addition to these sorts of memory problems, patients report a loss of isolated memories that occurs in an almost random fashion. It's almost as if some snippet of memory were edited out by the ECT. One of my patients went into her kitchen soon after ECT to bake her husband's favorite dessert, a pastry that she had made for years without a recipe, only to discover that she didn't have the recipe in her head anymore. As you might suspect, these kinds of memory problems are almost impossible to pick up on tests, and so despite many years of memory research on ECT patients it has been difficult to quantify very precisely the effect of ECT on these long-term memories. Another factor that confuses the issue is the effect that severe depression has on memory. Several studies indicate that complaints of memory problems after ECT correlate better with the severity of the patient's depression than with how they do on memory tests.[4] Unilateral ECT appears to reduce sharply the number of memory complaints.[5]

Although many patients report no memory problems whatsoever after ECT, and most who do report problems say that their memory problems are temporary and minor, there are a very few who report that their memory has never been quite the same. My impression is that memory problems are not significant difficulties for my patients, the vast majority of whom are grateful that such an effective treatment as ECT is available to them.

The mechanism by which ECT works continues to be profoundly mysterious. During seizure activity, the neurons of the brain fire simultaneously and rhythmically, and there is a massive discharge of many neurotransmitters. We used to compare ECT to cardiac defibrillation: just as applying a current to the heart muscle "resets" abnormal rhythms in cardiac muscle, perhaps ECT "resets" rhythmic discharges in the brain in some way. But newer work seems to indicate that, as with other treatments for bipolar disorder, the effect occurs at the level of the individual neurons. Animal experimentation indicates that ECT, like lithium, affects G proteins within the neurons. It may be that ECT, like lithium, works on the neuronal "tuning" mechanisms, the G protein/second-messenger system discussed in chapter 5.

ECT for Bipolar Disorder

ECT can be thought of as a symptomatic treatment for both phases of bipolar disorder: although it can quickly interrupt an episode of depression or mania, it does not have a long-term effect as a mood stabilizer (a *symptomatic* treatment treats *symptoms* but not the underlying disease process). Medication treatment will still be necessary to sustain the benefit of ECT and to keep the patient's mood state stable after the treatments are finished.

Typically, when the decision is made to give a course of ECT, all medications are stopped. (Sedative medications often shorten and otherwise interfere with the ECT "seizure," and so do the anticonvulsant mood stabilizers—they are anticonvulsants, after all! Lithium, meanwhile, seems to make patients more prone to episodes of confusion after their treatments.)

ECT is generally considered to be the most effective antidepressant treatment available. Naturally, it should be a treatment consideration whenever a bipolar patient continues to be severely depressed despite antidepressant medication treatment. It is also *rapidly* effective. Often, patients are dramatically improved after just three or four treatments—that is, after five to seven days. Severely suicidal patients or those who have stopped eating and drinking and are in danger of malnutrition and dehydration—any patients for whom profound depression has become an imminently life-threatening illness—are candidates for ECT. Pregnancy is also considered to be an indication for use of ECT to treat bipolar depression because of the risk most mood-stabilizing medications pose to the fetus.[6] Because depression can be highly resistant to antidepressant medications and also very dangerous in the elderly, ECT is frequently recommended as a first-line treatment for severe depression for older people as well. Depressed bipolar patients who receive ECT can become slightly hypomanic. When this occurs, obviously it's time to stop the treatments. Unlike the antidepressants, however, ECT does not seem to increase the cycling of the illness.[7]

ECT is also a highly effective treatment for mania. A 1994 review in the *American Journal of Psychiatry* of fifty years' experience of the use of ECT for treating mania found that it provided complete symptom remission or marked improvement in 80 percent of the manic patients studied. Many of the patients in these studies had failed to respond to many other available treatments—making this success rate all the more impressive.[8] ECT seems to work more quickly in mania than in depression. One study found that patients recovered after an average of six treatments, about half the usual requirement for the treatment of depression.[9] Severely manic patients whose highly agitated state becomes physically dangerous are obvious candidates for ECT, as are pregnant manic patients.

ECT is a valuable therapeutic tool for any bipolar patient who is very sick and seems to be getting sicker despite aggressive treatment with medication. It is also helpful for that small group of bipolar patients whom I call "brittle." These are patients, often with a rapid-cycling illness, who are poorly responsive to mood stabilizers and prone to adverse effects of other medications as well. They seem to start having manic symptoms if they so much as hold a Prozac capsule in their hand, but they crash into severe depression only days after getting a bit of relief from agitated mania with huge doses of antipsychotic medications; medications seem to do them more harm than good. Patients who have been either manic or severely depressed for months often have a dramatic response to ECT after everything else has failed, and once ECT has treated their acute symptoms, they can go on to have sustained periods of normal mood on medication.

ECT is perhaps the most effective treatment there is for severe depression and severe mania, and it often works more quickly than medications.[10] If you're beginning to wonder why ECT isn't used more often in bipolar disorder, you're in very good company. It is certainly much more complicated to go through general anaesthesia two or three times a week for two to four weeks than it is to take medication, but ECT may well still be underutilized, especially for patients sick enough to need hospitalization. We also know that bipolar depression can be less responsive to medication treatment, and there is the risk of antidepressants accelerating the cycling of bipolar illness. These facts make the use of ECT for severe bipolar depression even more compelling.

Transcranial Magnetic Stimulation

Transcranial magnetic stimulation (TMS) is a new experimental therapeutic technique similar to ECT that appears to be effective in treating mood disorders. TMS is currently a research technique only, but preliminary results with it are very encouraging. The great advantage of TMS over ECT is that TMS is much simpler to administer: no seizure activity is induced by the treatment, and therefore no anaesthesia is necessary.

This novel technique takes advantage of a principle of electromagnetism called *induction* to deliver an electrical stimulus to the brain without applying electrical energy to the scalp (as in ECT). During TMS treatments, a magnetic coil is held against the scalp, and the magnetic field that develops in the coil causes electrical current to flow through nearby neurons within the skull. No electricity passes through the skull, as in ECT; rather, the magnetic field "induces" a tiny electrical current in the underlying brain tissue. Since the electrical current that is generated in the brain tissue by TMS is so small, a seizure does not occur; thus, no anaesthesia is necessary. Pulses of magnetic energy are delivered over a period of about twenty minutes while the patient simply sits in a chair, awake and alert throughout the whole procedure. Oth-

FIGURE 10-1 Transcranial magnetic stimulation

er than some soreness from muscle stimulation, there appear to be no side effects of any kind.[11]

TMS has been used for a number of years to do brain mapping. The mapping of motor areas of the brain involves stimulating an area and then measuring electrical activity in the muscles controlled by that area. Stimulating a sensory area of the brain can cause a person to feel tingling in the part of the body that sends sensory nerves to that area. Sophisticated TMS techniques are also being used to study language functions and the organization of complex movements as well.

It is possible to give a placebo TMS treatment, making it easier to do valid research on the efficacy of TMS in depression. (A true placebo-controlled study of ECT would mean giving two groups of patients anaesthesia but giving the electrical stimulus only to patients in one of the groups. Risking anaesthesia to receive a fake ECT treatment is something few people would volunteer for, and ethically it is a rather dubious idea.) When the TMS coil is applied to the scalp at a slightly different angle from that normally used to give treatments, it does not cause electrical current to flow through the brain tissue and thus will not have the usual TMS effect. However, because stimulation of the muscles still occurs, the slight muscle soreness associated with the treatment occurs as well, and research subjects will have no way of knowing whether they are getting a sham treatment or the real thing. This makes the all important double-blind placebo-controlled studies fairly easy to do.

As we shall see in chapter 18, various studies indicate that the left prefrontal lobes of the brain are less active than normal in depression. This finding has led researchers to try TMS treatments on depressed patients by stimulating the left prefrontal lobes. Early results have been very promising. One of the first studies on TMS in the treatment of depression appeared in the *American Journal of Psychiatry* in 1997.[12] In this study from the National Institutes of Mental Health, twelve patients received twenty two-second TMS stimulations over a period of twenty minutes every weekday for two weeks. Either before or after the two weeks of therapy, the patients were given two weeks of "sham" treatments (the placebo), during which the TMS coil was held at an angle that would not cause brain tissue stimulation. The patients were tested for depressive symptoms by trained investigators using a standardized questionnaire. Neither the patients nor the investigators giving the mood questionnaire knew whether the patients were receiving real or sham TMS (making the study *double* blind). There was a statistically significant mood improvement in these patients after the real TMS treatments, but not after the sham treatments. Several patients continued TMS after the completion of the study and experienced even further clinical improvement in their depressive symptoms. In several studies, depressed patients with drug-resistant depression showed improvement after TMS.[13]

TMS is in its infancy. The strength of the magnetic stimulation that is most beneficial, the exact placement of the coil, the number of treatments, and the duration of therapy are all under investigation at various centers around the world. Will TMS, like ECT, be effective in bipolar depression as well as in unipolar depression? How about in mania? These and many other questions remain to be answered.

Perhaps the biggest unanswered question is, How does TMS work? It has always been thought that the seizure is the necessary therapeutic factor in ECT. Does TMS work in a different way? Or is TMS some kind of "gentler" ECT that works by a similar mechanism but without causing a seizure? (If the TMS coil is made to generate a strong enough magnetic field, a seizure can indeed be triggered with this technique, perhaps suggesting the latter explanation.)

It is clear, however, that TMS is a very promising development in the treatment of mood disorders and may open up a whole new array of treatment options.

CHAPTER 11

Counseling and Psychotherapy

ALTHOUGH MEDICAL TREATMENTS SUCH AS PHARMACEUTICALS ARE the foundation of the treatment of bipolar disorder, counseling and psychotherapy are important, perhaps indispensable additional therapeutic interventions for this illness. Some people still picture psychotherapy as something that happens in a richly paneled, dimly lit office where a bearded psychiatrist sits taking notes in a high-backed leather chair behind a patient lying on a couch who is trying to remember what he or she dreamed about last night. Or perhaps they think of talk-radio therapists, dispensing sound-bite-sized advice to the lovelorn and lonely between car commercials on the AM dial. Well, all this is psychotherapy of a sort, though it's not usually the sort of therapy that does people with bipolar disorder much good.

But many types of counseling and therapy *are* enormously helpful in bipolar disorder. If you've read this book to this point, you've already had several hours of therapy of a kind. You've allowed an objective but sympathetic individual with knowledge and experience about mental illness and psychological processes (that's me) to present facts about bipolar disorder to increase your understanding of the illness. This understanding has, I hope, helped you make sense of your thoughts and feelings about this problem as it affects you, and helped prepare you to make decisions based on knowledge rather than on emotions such as fear of or anger about the illness. This is, in large measure, what therapy is all about: not interpreting dreams, not simply doling out advice, and certainly not supplying all the answers, but providing good information, objective feedback, and solid encouragement in a supportive, confidential setting.

Brain and Mind

In chapter 2 I described how manic-depressive illness came to be called a "functional" psychiatric illness in the early twentieth century. After the discovery of the biological causes of mental illnesses like general paresis (central nervous system syphilis) and cretinism (mental retardation due to thyroid deficiency), psychiatric illnesses came to be divided into two categories: *organic* and *functional*. Organic psychiatric illnesses were "real" illnesses, caused by germs or abnormal hormone levels or something else that could be seen under a microscope or measured in a blood test. In functional illnesses, on the other hand, it was assumed that there wasn't anything wrong with brain functioning in a physical sense. Patients with manic-depressive illness or schizophrenia were having some kind of abnormal reaction to life events.

The question then became, Why do some people have these very abnormal reactions while others do not? It was at this point that the attempt to understand and treat these illnesses turned away from medicine and toward psychology. Sigmund Freud spent his lifetime treating and trying to understand patients who were unhappy in their relationships, disappointed in themselves for the choices they had made, perhaps confused and anxious about decisions they were facing. Freud and his followers developed a large and sophisticated system for understanding human behavior based on understanding childhood development. They developed treatments that basically consisted of helping patients understand themselves better, let go of grudges, resentments, and fears rooted in their past, and learn better, more mature coping mechanisms. This approach has come to be called *dynamic* psychology or psychiatry and is based on the belief that mental life is best understood as a dynamic interplay between emotions and intellect, present circumstances and unconscious memories of past experiences, and many other psychological factors.

Although this approach was extremely successful in helping people with a wide variety of problems and symptoms, practitioners of dynamic psychotherapy soon discovered that it didn't make much of an impact on the symptoms of illnesses like schizophrenia or bipolar disorder. These patients were thought by most traditional psychotherapists to be too disturbed or too immature or their families too dysfunctional for them to benefit from therapy. Then a revolution occurred: lithium, chlorpromazine, and other effective medications for "functional" illnesses came along. In the 1970s, persons with bipolar disorder and schizophrenia left the many therapists who had been blaming them and their families for their illnesses and made tracks for a new kind of doctor: the biological psychiatrist, the pharmacotherapist, someone who would treat them like real people dealing with a "real" illness. For a time there was a kind of schism in American psychiatry between those who believed that dynamic psychology best explained mental illnesses and those who believed that biology was the key that would unlock the mysteries of psychiatric disorders.

When I was interviewing for psychiatric training programs in the mid-1970s, this biological psychiatry/dynamic psychiatry split was at its most pronounced. Many university medical center departments of psychiatry proudly identified themselves to me as either "biological" or "psychodynamic" in their approach. Usually each camp denigrated the other: psychodynamic psychiatry was "touchy-feely" soft science based more on nineteenth-century literary theory than on medicine; biological psychiatrists were "pill-pushers" who didn't even talk to their patients and had no appreciation for the human experience. But a few departments of psychiatry—Johns Hopkins' was one— were teaching their residents that mental experiences were neither a series of chemical reactions nor simply a collection of dynamically interrelated thoughts and feelings, but both. We learned at Hopkins that people with bipolar disorder are still people, still subject to disappointments and loss, to relationship problems and blows to their self-esteem. To regard their moods as just the expression of so many chemicals to be fine-tuned with more chemicals was to do them a great disservice. (Maybe that's how I came to dislike that phrase "chemical imbalance.") Fortunately this schism has now healed for the most part, and even the most ardent biological psychiatrists understand that psychodynamic understanding of the patient is *always* important. There are also many kinds of psychological therapies now, and most do not involve the psychoanalytic couch.

Although there is certainly a place for dynamic psychotherapy in modern psychiatry—*including* traditional Freudian psychoanalysis and the psychoanalytic couch—the variety of available psychological treatments has broadened tremendously in the past twenty-five years or so. Sophisticated techniques have been developed that work for particular kinds of problems. Some involve individual sessions with a therapist, others a group setting. Some are focused on a particular problem, such as marital or family difficulties, others on a particular symptom, such as depression or panic attacks. Some are designed to last only a few sessions; others are more open-ended. Some are not "therapy" in the traditional sense at all: support groups, made up of individuals who offer guidance and support to each other, don't even include a "therapist." Moreover, a lot of research has been done on which psychological treatments work best for which problems. The prescription of a particular kind of counseling or therapy for a particular kind of problem is often backed up by as much research as is the prescription of a particular medication.

What Can Therapy Do?

No one today would even think to recommend counseling or therapy as the only treatment for bipolar disorder; to do so would constitute malpractice. But because we have highly effective medications for this illness, some doctors, and perhaps many more patients, want to turn away from counseling and therapy altogether and approach the illness as a purely "chemical" problem that has a purely "chemical" solution. This is a mistake, for several reasons.

First of all, the diagnosis of bipolar disorder is almost always a traumatic event, not only for patients but for their family members as well. In addition to the emotional turmoil that is the symptom of the illness itself, there is an emotional reeling that results from coming face to face with fears about how this diagnosis will affect one's life. Vaguely familiar terms like *manic-depression* and all too familiar terms like *mental illness* conjure up all sorts of confused and confusing ideas and feelings. "Why has this happened to me?" (or perhaps "This *can't* be happening to me!") and "My life will never be the same" and "Whose fault is this?" are only some of the thoughts and questions that start spinning through the minds of people affected by this diagnosis. Remember that I described therapy as "providing good information, objective feedback, and solid encouragement in a supportive, confidential setting." It becomes obvious, doesn't it, that this kind of psychological treatment is going to be necessary and very helpful. Some research suggests that the first year after a diagnosis of bipolar disorder is a crucial time for persons with the disorder, and that the education, support, and encouragement that psychotherapy provides are very important in making treatment successful in the long term.[1]

Another traumatic event that persons with bipolar disorder face all too frequently is relapse. The management of bipolar disorder is still far from perfect, and despite everyone's best efforts, relapse can and does occur. Many patients feel that they're "back to square one"; they blame themselves or their medication or their doctor; they become angry, disappointed, discouraged, and confused about what to do next. Again, counseling helps the person put things back into perspective, get over the setback, and move on. I shall discuss individual therapy in more detail later in this chapter.

Group Psychotherapy

Psychotherapy can be very effective in a group setting. In group therapy a therapist meets with a group of patients rather than with only one individual. The worry I often hear expressed by patients for whom group therapy is recommended is that they don't want to "sit around listening to other people's problems" week after week. But no group therapist worth his or her salt is going to let the group deteriorate into a "pity party"; instead, he or she will guide the group members onto the track of learning from, and helping solve, one another's problems—not just ventilating about them. And an excellent way to become a better problem solver is to see how other people are managing, or failing, to solve their own problems.

In traditional group psychotherapy, groups are usually made up of persons with a variety of problems. In the treatment of bipolar disorder, however, *homogeneous* groups (groups composed exclusively of persons with bipolar disorder) have been studied more and have been shown to be effective. Several studies show that bipolar-disorder patients in group therapy have fewer relapses and improved productivity at work or school.[2] The research suggests that the shared aspect of the problems seems to be very important to the therapeutic experience. Persons with bipolar disorder who are in groups with other bipolar-disorder patients report that the practical advice they receive about living with the disorder is very helpful. Their understanding of the disorder, of how it affects their relationships and self-attitudes, is enhanced, and the guidance they receive from group members is perceived as very valuable.[3] This aspect of group therapy—sharing and learning from one another—is the basis of another type of "therapy," one that doesn't require a therapist: peer support groups. We shall discuss this helping format in chapter 20.

Individual Therapy for Depression

As we saw in several earlier chapters, available pharmaceutical treatments for the depressed phase of bipolar disorder are less than perfect by a long shot. The mood stabilizers are often not very good antidepressants, and antidepressant medications carry the risk of precipitating mania or accelerating the frequency of cycles. But psychotherapy has a proven track record in helping with depression and, as far as we can tell, has no risk of precipitating mania or of accelerating the course of bipolar disorder.

"Now wait a minute," I can hear you say, "I've been reading through this entire book that the moods of bipolar disorder are caused by abnormal brain chemistry, and now you want me to believe that psychotherapy can treat the depressive phase of bipolar disorder?" Well, perhaps "psychotherapy can treat the depressive phase of bipolar disorder" overstates the case a bit, but there is some research showing—by implication, at least—that it may be very helpful.

In the 1960s Dr. Aaron Beck and his colleagues developed a theory of and psychotherapeutic treatment for depression called *cognitive therapy*.[4] This type of psychotherapy has been researched more thoroughly than most others and has a proven track record in helping with symptoms of depression; in some studies—though not in others—it has been found to work as well as, even better than, antidepressant medication for some patients.[5]

The theory of cognitive therapy maintains that people who are chronically or frequently depressed have developed a somewhat distorted view of themselves and of the world and have adopted certain patterns of thinking and reacting that perpetuate their problems. This emphasis on thinking, or *cognition*, lends the theory and the therapy its name. As we saw in chapter 1, depressed persons tend (1) to think negatively about themselves, (2) to interpret their experiences in a negative way, and (3) to have a pessimistic view of the future. Cognitive theory calls this the "cognitive triad."[6] The theory further proposes that all this negative thinking causes a person to develop a repertoire of mental habits called "schemas"[7] or "negative automatic thoughts" that spring into action and reinforce the negative thinking.

John is a thirty-two-year-old computer specialist whose idea for a new project has just been turned down by his company. He comes to his therapy session and brings along a lengthy handwritten critique of the project that the senior vice-president of his division left behind after coming by John's cubicle to tell him that the project had been turned down.

"You see, I should have known better than to take on that big a project. The senior vice-president, no less, comes by with the bad news. 'Better luck next time,' she said. Now I'm never going to move up in this company."

"Why do you say that?" I asked.

"If someone that high up thinks I'm incompetent, I'm done for. That's the last time I bother trying something I'm not cut out for."

"Did she say she thought you were incompetent?"

"Well, no, of course not."

"I see. This vice-president doesn't tell people what she thinks."

"Oh, no, that's not true at all. She's got a reputation for coming right out with her opinions about things."

"But she treats you differently from everyone else?"

John began to get a little annoyed. "Well, I wouldn't think so, but how should I know? I'd never talked with her before."

"What do you make of that?" I asked. "The fact that she came in person to give you the news about your proposal?"

"Well, I did think it was unusual."

"Could it mean she was impressed with some aspects of your proposal and wanted to meet you?"

"Well, I suppose that's possible."

I continued reinterpreting John's negative assumptions: "And how about the handwritten critique?"

"It was really negative," John went on glumly. "She went through every point and shot them down one by one."

"When had you sent the proposal to Ms. Kaiser? How long did she have to look at it?"

"Oh, I didn't send it to Kaiser; she's over the whole division. I had sent it to Bob Rodney, my team leader. I guess he sent it up to her, but I don't know how long she spent with it."

"Well, she must have spent several hours with it if she gave you back such a carefully organized critique. Don't you think?"

"Yeah, I guess she wouldn't have taken all that time and trouble if she had thought it was worthless."

"And your team leader must have thought it had some potential if he sent the proposal to *his* boss. Have you asked him for some feedback?"

"No, I assumed he'd be down on me for it, too."

"But do you see how your negative assumption stopped you from checking in with your team leader and prevented you from getting what could have been positive feedback and encouragement from him?"

"I see what you mean. If I hadn't jumped to conclusions, I might have gotten some positive strokes."

John is down on his talents and assumes everybody else is, too. In situations that can be interpreted many different ways, both positive and negative, he tends to go for the negative rather than seek alternative positive explanations. This in turn sometimes causes him to do things that reinforce his negative thinking, and the vicious cycle repeats itself. This might seem to be a trivial example, but it's not difficult to come up with a number of negative schemas that people with bipolar disorder are prone to:

Negative: "I got manic even though I was taking my lithium. It doesn't matter what I do. What's the use?"

Realistic: "Relapses occur even with medication. It might have been much worse and lasted much longer if I hadn't been on medication. Perhaps this new medication will be more effective for me."

Negative: "Everyone will be avoiding me when I go back to work. No one wants to work with a mentally ill person.

Realistic: "Some people might avoid me at work, perhaps many at first. But when they see that I'm the same old me, they'll come around. And those who don't are people I don't want as friends anyway."

Cognitive-therapy techniques more specifically focused on bipolar disorder are being developed. Part of the treatment deals with the negative automatic thoughts that interfere with treatment with medication. For example, if a person with bipolar disorder is troubled by the negative automatic thought "Taking mood-stabilizing medication is a sign of personal weakness" every time he or she take a dose of lithium, he or she might be more likely to skip doses or stop taking the medication altogether. Cognitive therapy works on the psychological barriers to proper treatment by replacing automatic negative thoughts with realistic ones.[8]

Cognitive therapy has been proven to be effective in the treatment of depression. Clearly it cannot replace medication treatment for bipolar disorder, but perhaps more than any other form of psychotherapy, it holds great promise for bipolar patients.

New Psychotherapies for Bipolar Disorder

For many years psychiatrists and the therapists who work with them in treating patients with bipolar disorder have had a sort of intuition that there are fewer relapses among patients who understand their illness and their treatment better, who work on learning to cope better with the stresses and difficulties that everybody faces, and whose family members are also informed and supportive. Psychiatrists have also observed that life stresses, difficult relationships at home, and even disruptions of sleep cycles seem to bring on symptoms and to impact the course of the illness. Often, though, they find it hard to persuade patients—and sometimes hard to persuade themselves, perhaps—that a course of traditional psychotherapy is what's needed.

Psychiatrists have done their best to spend time with patients and their families answering their questions about bipolar disorder and its treatments; trying to persuade patients with marital problems to get marital therapy and patients with job problems to get career counseling; and encouraging them to learn about stress management, watch their sleep habits, and steer clear of conflict and difficult situations whenever possible. But a lot of these interventions are time-consuming or expensive (or both), they are difficult to put into practice ("Steer clear of conflict? How do I do *that*, Doc?"), and until recently we have had only the impression that these are important interventions, with little hard data to back up our recommendations.

But now several research teams are developing treatment models of psychological therapy for bipolar patients that draw on these sorts of impressions. These models take into account the available research about the particular kinds of stresses that cause symptoms in bipolar patients, and they incorporate the experiences of clinicians who have treated many, many bipolar patients. These treatments emphasize things like patient and family education about the illness, stress management and conflict resolution, and close attention to the strains in family and marital relationships often caused by this illness in even the healthiest family units. These teams are testing their ideas with well-designed clinical research studies, and the results of these studies have been very encouraging. One or another or a combination of these therapies may well become standard recommendations for patients with bipolar disorder in the future.

These treatments differ from standard psychotherapy in several ways. Traditional psychotherapy is often unfocused and "exploratory"; the patient and the therapist work on the issues the patient identifies ("I want to learn to make better choices in my relationships"), and treatment is open-ended: the patient is in therapy as long as he or she finds it beneficial and has an issue to work on. These new treatments, however, are very focused. The focus varies slightly in the two current models: one focuses on family education and communication and the other on lifestyle regularization and stress management. In both kinds of treatment the therapist often acts more like a teacher or coach than a counselor, and the goals are to develop concrete solutions to real problems and to learn about and master new problem-solving techniques. Since the patient often doesn't bring "issues" to the therapy, there is a specified time course to the treatment; the main work of the treatment is "finished" within a certain time period, although there is a "maintenance" phase that can be indefinite.

Behavioral family management for bipolar disorder (BFM-BP) emphasizes the patient's family unit. It is a model that to some extent has grown out of research showing that patients with schizophrenia had more illness relapses if there were conflicts and stresses at home and within the family. This therapy works hard at family support. Educating the patient and his or her family members about the symptoms of bipolar disorder and its treatments is a priority, emphasizing that bipolar disorder is indeed an illness and that symptoms are not under voluntary control. Family sessions are held to identify difficulties and conflicts within the family unit—whether caused by the illness or by other, perhaps preexisting factors or situations. Conflict resolution and problem-solving techniques are presented and practiced, and healthy communication skills are developed through role playing and rehearsals.

Interpersonal and social rhythm therapy (IP/SRT) puts more emphasis on patients as individuals and on their "social rhythm." Based on the observation that sleep deprivation and other disruptions of body rhythms can bring on symptoms, this treatment emphasizes stability and stress management. It involves having patients track their mood states on a daily basis and also their daily routine with a sort of checklist of activities called the *social rhythm metric.*

In their sessions the patient and the therapist review these diaries and also the patient's "interpersonal inventory" (a list of the persons in the patient's social network) with an eye toward identifying conflicts and stresses in relationships. The therapist and the patient work on identifying emotional or physical stresses and factors in the environment that upset daily rhythms and emotional stability. The goal is to "find a healthy balance between daily rhythm stability, social activity, social stimulation and mood states."[9] Although it's still too soon to know the impact of IP/SRT on the course of bipolar disorder over time, early results of the research indicate that IP/SRT patients made more healthy lifestyle changes and showed greater stability in daily routines and rhythms than a control group of patients did.[10]

The research on BFM-BP and IP/SRT is still going on, and definitive results are a few years off. But for the first time research on the psychotherapeutic treatment of bipolar disorder is becoming just as scientific as research on the medication treatment of the disorder. It's only a matter of time before these results and further refinements of these therapies point the way to even better and more specific psychotherapy and counseling techniques for bipolar disorder.

"Traditional" Individual Psychotherapy

I hope I haven't given you the impression that traditional psychotherapy isn't useful for patients with bipolar disorder. Quite the contrary. Kay Jamison has written:

> At this point in my existence, I cannot imagine leading a normal life without both taking lithium and having had the benefits of psychotherapy. Lithium prevents my seductive but disastrous highs, diminishes my depressions . . . and makes psychotherapy possible. But, ineffably, psychotherapy *heals*. It makes some sense of the confusion, reins in the terrifying thoughts and feelings, returns some control and hope and possibility of learning from it all.[11]

So far in this chapter we've talked about "situational" supportive counseling focused around episodes of illness, either the first or a relapse, with the goal of helping patients deal with the acute stresses of diagnosis, hospitalization, reintegration back into their job, or other specific issues related to an episode of illness. We've discussed the cognitive therapy of depression, a course of treatment that might be recommended for chronic or smoldering depressive symptoms that medication alone doesn't seem to quite take care of. In the last section we discussed some new therapies that aim to teach patients and their families how to smooth out the bumpy spots in their relationships, improve communication and conflict resolution skills, and regularize their social rhythms. These treatments are perhaps more preventive than the others and might be thought of as providing psychological immunization against future problems as well as ways of dealing with present ones.

What, then, of traditional psychotherapy? By *traditional psychotherapy* I mean individual meetings with a therapist, usually over an extended period of time (months or years), in which the person in treatment discusses his or her past and present experiences and feelings with the goal of self-understanding, self-acceptance, and personal growth. (*Dynamic* or *insight-oriented psychotherapy* is the same thing.) Disappointments and accomplishments, affections and enmities, fears, inspirations, passions, and worries—all are, as psychotherapists are fond of saying, "grist for the mill" of therapy. Patient and therapist will, of course, talk about symptoms like sadness and anxiety too, but traditional therapy sees symptoms as indicators of underlying conflicts rather than as the focus of treatment in and of themselves. Traditional psychotherapy emphasizes exploration of the *meaning* of symptoms, the development of self-awareness and maturity.

So when would we recommend traditional psychotherapy to a person with bipolar disorder? For what types of problems would it be helpful? Basically, for the same types of problems that people without bipolar disorder go to therapists for: dealing with psychological traumas and setbacks—past and present—that cause understandable feelings of sadness, anger, or anxiety, or thought patterns, self-attitudes, and interpersonal styles that disrupt a person's ability to be happy in relationships, effective at work, carefree in play, and confident about making decisions about the future. Sounds like a tall order, doesn't it? Well, of course it is. That is why psychotherapists often study and train in their profession for almost as many years as physicians train in theirs. That is why people are sometimes in therapy for months, even for years, at a time. That is why psychotherapy is such an intense, powerful experience and the therapeutic relationship between patient and therapist a unique one.

Bipolar patients will often have had more than their share of setbacks and psychological traumas—both past and present. Because it is a genetic illness, persons with bipolar disorder often have had difficult, even traumatic childhoods. Perhaps a parent was afflicted with the illness, perhaps he or she could not or would not receive proper treatment, and the child may have suffered disruptions to family life, periods of poverty or homelessness, perhaps even physical or emotional abuse. Psychotherapy can be enormously beneficial in helping people face and work through their difficult pasts, let go of the anger, resentment, and fear that often comes out of these experiences, and move on with their lives.

The fact that a person has bipolar disorder can make ordinary life decisions seem complex and important life decisions seem overwhelming. There is no better way of dealing with these sorts of anxieties and apprehensions than traditional psychotherapy. I remember a young woman who came to see me for a routine medication-monitoring appointment when I was working in the very busy medication clinic of a community mental-health center, a clinical setting in which patients were scheduled every twenty minutes. "I've been dating a man for several months now, and I think he might ask me to marry him," she told me. She looked worried. "I haven't told him about my illness. I don't know what to tell him. How do you think I should handle this?" I stared at her helplessly for a moment and panicked just a little when I heard the nurse slipping the chart of the next patient into the bin outside the interviewing-room door. I hope I didn't sound as rushed as I felt when I tried to convince her that the situation raised an enormous number of complex issues. How, when, where, why, and with whom she discussed her diagnosis was going to need much more than one—or a dozen—twenty-minute appointments with me to get into, let alone resolve.

I doubt very much that this was the first time this young woman had been confused about what to tell someone about her diagnosis. Perhaps she had muddled through other situations at work, at church, or in her neighborhood, maybe saying nothing about her diagnosis because of feelings of shame, or maybe blurting out too much about herself and then feeling vulnerable and exposed. Perhaps being diagnosed with bipolar disorder reactivated feelings she had struggled with in childhood or adolescence about being teased for being too fat or too skinny—or perhaps, more likely in a bipolar patient, too "hyper" or "weird." I was sure that since we had discussed the fact that bipolar disorder is a genetic illness, a possible marriage proposal raised questions in her mind about having children who might be affected by the disorder. How had the diagnosis affected her identity as a potential parent, as a woman? Or perhaps none of these issues needed to be explored but instead other, completely different ones. Well, all these things are what good old-fashioned once-a-week "How do you feel about that?" psychotherapy is all about.

Psychotherapy in Bipolar Disorder: Is It Really Necessary?

All the psychiatrists I know talk about how much time they spend trying to persuade their bipolar patients to supplement their medication treatment with some form of therapy. I think there is a vast variety of reasons why persons with bipolar disorder are reluctant to do so. Some patients have made uneasy peace with taking medication for a psychiatric illness (or, as they might put it to themselves, only a "chemical imbalance"), but they see going to psychotherapy as confirmation of the "mental" aspect of their "mental illness." But if you think about it, the treatment of even the most "medical" of medical illnesses—heart disease, say, or a ruptured lumbar disk—usually requires nonmedical interventions, and sometimes these turn out to be just as important as the pharmaceutical or even surgical interventions prescribed by the doctor. The patient with diabetes would hardly regard staying on a healthy diet and watching his or her weight as unnecessary adjuncts to the management of the illness with insulin injections. The recovering coronary-bypass surgery patient wouldn't think to ignore the physician's recommendation for a cardiac-hardening exercise program. Would anyone have an operation for lumbar disk problems and skip the physical therapy sessions afterward? I don't think so.

We know that chronic psychological stresses make a whole variety of physical illnesses more difficult to treat: asthma, high blood pressure, irritable bowel syndrome. Psychological stresses will make mood-disorder symptoms more difficult to control as well.

The research results on the psychotherapeutic treatments of bipolar disorder aren't all in, so we can't yet specify particular therapies for a particular duration of time for particular mood syndromes. But the available research and many years of clinical experience indicate that psychotherapy and counseling have been enormously helpful to countless patients with bipolar disorder. If a particular type of therapy or counseling is available, is affordable, and has been recommended by the physician or treatment team, persons with bipolar disorder owe it to themselves to take advantage of the unique healing powers of these marvelous therapeutic techniques.

The Psychiatrist-Psychotherapist: An Extinct Species?

You have probably noticed that throughout this chapter I usually refer to the psychiatrist and the psychotherapist as two different individuals. Unfortunately this has become the rule rather than the exception in American psychiatry for most patients. It would, of course, be preferable for all sorts of reasons for the person prescribing medication and the person doing psychotherapy to be one and the same individual. But for a variety of complicated reasons, most people with bipolar disorder will see a psychiatrist for medication management and a nonphysician therapist—often a social worker or psychologist—for therapy. Some of the reasons for this are the changes in medication management of bipolar disorder that have come about with the development of new medications; there are now so many different pharmaceuticals used in psychiatry that staying skilled in their use has become more and more time-consuming. Perhaps even more significantly, as more and more effective medications become available for more psychiatric problems, more and more patients want (and need) to see a psychiatrist for their treatment. There simply aren't enough psychiatrists to do medication management and therapy too, especially in busy clinics. Since medical school and psychiatric training take longer and cost more than the training required to become a psychotherapist, psychiatrists are usually more expensive than other professionals. When the administrator of a busy clinic or HMO is looking to staff the organization's mental-health program, "split" treatment—psychiatric treatment split between a psychiatrist for medication management and a nonphysician therapist for psychotherapy or counseling—means more cost-effective treatment for patients.

The superior cost-effectiveness of "split" treatment allows so many more patients to receive psychiatric treatment so much more cheaply that it's difficult to envision a return to the days when psychiatrists did therapy and prescribed medications, too. Fortunately there are excellent training programs for clinical social workers, psychologists, and counseling professionals that are producing superb psychotherapists. And as we have seen in this chapter, psychotherapy is becoming more specialized, too. It has become nearly impossible to be an expert therapist and at the same time an expert psychopharmacologist. For all of these reasons, the medication management and the therapy of the person with bipolar disorder will usually be handled by two professionals rather than one.

CHAPTER 12

Treatment Approaches in Bipolar Disorder

THE BASIC CAUSE OF BIPOLAR DISORDER REMAINS UNKNOWN. TREAT-
ment approaches have been stumbled upon more or less by accident—as with
the discovery of the therapeutic effects of lithium—and although they have
been refined by decades of experience, they are still largely what physicians call
empirical. This means that the treatment is based on experience—on therapeutic results rather than on a true understanding of the mechanism of the
disease or symptom in question.[1]

Therapeutic Results as a Guide to Treatment

Although we have a tremendous amount of experience in the use of pharmaceuticals to treat bipolar disorder and have data on their effectiveness in
large groups of patients, the treatment of individual patients with bipolar disorder is often guided by treatment results rather than by the kinds of hard data
physicians use to treat other illnesses. What do I mean by this? Let me explain
by referring to a very different kind of illness, pneumonia.

A young man is rushed to an emergency room with a high fever, a pain in
his chest, difficulty breathing, and a congested cough. The doctor orders a
chest x-ray. A specimen of the young man's sputum is rushed off to the laboratory, and a tiny droplet is spread on a microscope slide, immersed in a special dye called a Gram stain, and examined under the microscope. More tiny
droplets of sputum are spread over the surface of several flat dishes (Petri dishes) containing mixtures of proteins and other nutrients that various bacteria

are known to grow on. On one of the dishes are a number of little paper disks that have been soaked in different antibiotics.

The lab results start coming in. The young man's chest x-ray shows that one of the lobes of his right lung is filled with fluid. The Gram stain reveals that his phlegm is loaded with bacteria aligned in pairs and linked into short chains: the pneumococcus. The diagnosis is clear: pneumococcal pneumonia. The doctor starts the young man on penicillin, an antibiotic known to be effective against most strains of pneumococcus, and within eight hours his fever is dropping. The dose of penicillin and the length of time the young man will need to take it have been determined by years of experience, calculated to the milligram and to the hour.

In a day or so the lab reports that the Petri dish containing the pneumococcus' favorite food is full of colonies of bacteria that other, more sophisticated techniques now definitely confirm as pneumococcus. The best news of all is that in the dish containing the little disks of antibiotics, there is a wide halo around the penicillin disk: the penicillin is effectively inhibiting the growth of the strain of bacteria causing this particular case of pneumonia. This means that the young man does not have a pneumonia caused by a penicillin-resistant bug, and his speedy recovery is assured.

The doctor treating this young man had quite a bit of hard data on which to base his or her treatment decisions. The x-ray indicated that this was probably a typical bacterial lobar pneumonia rather than viral pneumonia, tuberculosis, or any of a number of other conditions with similar symptoms but different pictures on x-ray. Also—and very important for prognostic purposes—the x-ray indicated that only one lobe was involved. With the results of the Gram stain, the likely identity of the bacterial culprit was determined within minutes, allowing the quick choice of a drug known to be effective most of the time against this type of germ. The identity of the bacterial culprit was solidly confirmed several days later when it grew in the culture dish and could be further tested. Most important, the lab results showed which drug would work against the germ causing the problem in this particular patient.

On the other hand, when a patient with manic symptoms comes into the ER, there are no tests to order—just the eyes and ears and experience of the psychiatrist. Fortunately, or perhaps unfortunately, full-blown mania is often an unmistakable diagnosis, and effective antimanic drugs are readily available. But what of the person who comes to the office and says "I'm depressed" or complains of "mood swings." There are many more diagnostic possibilities. We know that antidepressant medications can sometimes make a patient with bipolar symptoms worse. How is a physician to know whether or not a person who comes in with symptoms of depression will turn out to have a bipolar illness? There are hints, of course, such as family history, but wouldn't it be fantastic if we could order a test for bipolar disorder before considering an antidepressant for a person who is having symptoms of depression? But we can't. And how about the treatment once the acute symptoms have been controlled? Emil Kraepelin described some patients who had a remission of their bipolar symptoms that lasted for decades (apparently quite rarely, but he observed them nevertheless). Do we prescribe a mood stabilizer for a patient who might not get sick again for ten or even twenty years? Wouldn't it be great if we could stop the medication after a period of time and have the patient come in every couple of months for some kind of scan that could pick up changes in brain chemistry before symptoms became apparent? That way the patient would take medication only as it became necessary. Sometimes patients respond to one mood stabilizer but not another, or to a combination of two mood stabilizers but to neither one when used alone. How to choose? Wouldn't it be fantastic if we could take a blood sample and look for some kind of chemical reaction around little paper disks soaked with lithium or Prozac in a Petri dish to help us choose effective medications for a particular patient?

Unfortunately at the present moment we don't have any blood tests, scans, or other laboratory tests to make the treatment approach to bipolar disorder as informed and logical as the approach can be in some other illnesses. Therefore the approach to the treatment of bipolar illness can be discussed only in general terms. Patients are started on the medications that have been proven effective in many patients with similar symptoms, and if their symptoms are not effectively treated, other medications are tried.

So the bad news is that we can't test for bipolar disorder or pick from among similar agents knowing beforehand which one of them will work best. There is unfortunately a lot of "trial and error" and "wait and see" when it comes to prescribing medications for a specific patient. This can be tremendously frustrating for all involved—for the patient, of course, and for family members, and, yes, for the physician, too.

But the good news is that more and better medications are becoming available all the time. Twenty years ago there was only one mood-stabilizing medication, lithium. Ten years ago there were three. Now we have at least five and several more on the way. There are easily twice as many antidepressants on the market as there were only fifteen years ago. The newer antipsychotic medications have fewer side effects, and some seem to have mood-stabilizing properties that the older agents lacked.

Despite what you might see in the movies, electroconvulsive therapy is one of the safest medical procedures available—and probably underutilized in bipolar disorder. Transcranial magnetic stimulation may come to replace ECT if it delivers what it seems to be promising.

Don't forget counseling and psychotherapy. Research has proven how very important this unique treatment is in controlling the symptoms of mood disorders. More effective therapy programs for bipolar disorder are being refined by researchers with studies as rigorous as those used to evaluate any pharmaceutical.

And I haven't even talked about light therapy and sleep manipulation yet (that's coming in chapter 16). Researchers have discovered that exposure to bright light and changes in sleep patterns can help regulate mood and perhaps help medications work better and faster.

A Few Principles of Treatment

Every once in a while one of the medical journals publishes a "treatment algorithm" for bipolar disorder. An algorithm is a step-by-step procedure for solving a specified problem with mathematical precision. A treatment algorithm for acute mania might look something like this:

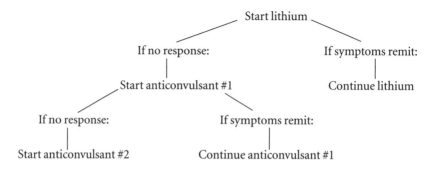

Start lithium

If no response: If symptoms remit:

Start anticonvulsant #1   Continue lithium

If no response: If symptoms remit:

Start anticonvulsant #2   Continue anticonvulsant #1

Well, you get the idea. I don't pay much attention to treatment algorithms anymore. They don't usually tell me anything new about medications, and their "if this happens, then do that" approach never captures the myriad manifestations of the disorder, the inevitable twists and turns of the world of real treatment and real patients, not to mention the specific situations and needs of the individual. That said, there are several principles of treatment that do serve patients (and their physicians) well. You'll notice, however, that these principles don't include many specifics about medications.

With so many powerful and effective medications available in psychiatry now, it's sometimes easy to become impatient when symptoms don't subside as quickly as one would wish. But in the treatment of mood disorders, a crucial principle to remember is to *take the long view.*

I saw Craig about two weeks after he had been discharged from a hospital in another city. He had been on a business trip and started to have fairly severe manic symptoms: insomnia, racing thoughts, angry irritability. He had been having good control of his symptoms on a mood stabilizer, but a series of high-stress job interviews in several different cities, jet lag, worry, and poor sleep had activated his illness, and he soon found himself hospitalized in a city several hundred miles from home.

He pulled a fistful of medication bottles out of his pocket and put them on the desk in my office. "I brought all these new medicines, but I have to admit, I've only been taking the lithium."

I picked up the bottles one by one: lithium, valproate, an antipsychotic, an anti-anxiety agent, and a sleeping pill.

"How long were you in the hospital?" I asked.

"Eight days."

"And you were discharged on *all* this?"

"That's right. I can't believe I really need all this. I was so drugged when my wife came to pick me up. I couldn't work for another week and a half. I think this is the first day I've felt safe to drive."

Craig's illness had always been very responsive to medications; it was hard for me to believe that all these medications had really been necessary. How had this happened?

When I asked Craig about his treatment in the hospital, a sadly familiar story emerged: a new medication had been added to the mix almost every other day while he was in the hospital. He was started on the antipsychotic medication as soon as he was admitted. Well, that wasn't unreasonable; I might have recommended that myself—for a while, at least. But when he didn't sleep well the next night, a sleeping pill was added. A few days later, when he mentioned that he had been worried about his finances lately, an anti-anxiety medication was added. After a week he told his doctor he was feeling less hyper but still not back to his usual self—so the valproate was added to the lithium. By the time he left the hospital, he wasn't complaining of mood problems anymore because he was too sedated to know *what* kind of mood he was in.

"Craig, you know I want you to call the clinic before you make any changes in your medication on your own," I said with a smile. "But I have to admit, in the end you did exactly what I would have recommended that you do. You certainly don't need all this."

Craig smiled back. "Well, great minds think alike—don't we?"

The medications we use to treat mood disorders usually take at least two weeks to have their full effect. When treating an episode of bipolar disorder, it usually doesn't make sense to change medications quickly. Even hospitalized patients are rarely well served by adding too many medications too quickly. And in patients having more minor mood symptoms, the four-week rule is a good one. I usually tell patients to try a medication for at least a month before they decide how it is working for them. (Intolerable side effects would, of course, cancel this advice—but even side effects usually get better with time, and sticking it out for at least a few days is often all that is needed.)

When a diagnosis of bipolar II or cyclothymic disorder is being considered, the time line should stretch out even more. The mood changes in these variations of bipolar disorder can sometimes be much more subtle than those of bipolar I. It may take three to six months of taking a mood stabilizer for its beneficial effects on a subtly unstable mood to become apparent.

In Craig's case it was the doctor who forgot to take the long view, but I think it's probably even easier for patients or their family members to fall into the trap of expecting results too quickly.

"Cindy's still having mood swings, Doctor," Jim said as he sat down beside his wife in the office. "The Depakote isn't working. Is there something else we can try?"

Jim and Cindy were a couple in their thirties. They had two small children, and Cindy usually cared for her attorney sister's little boy during the day as well as caring for her own.

Cindy was tense and quiet as her husband continued. "She's been on this medication for two weeks now, and things are no different. She started arguing with me about the television being too loud the other night, and when I tried to reason with her, she picked up the remote control and threw it at me. This has got to stop."

"What do you think, Cindy?" I asked. "Do you think the medication has helped any?"

"Well, I'm not sure, but I think maybe it has."

"Well, I'm sure it hasn't," said Jim. "The night before the remote incident she—"

"Jim," I said, "it's much too early to be sure about anything yet. Cindy's only been taking the Depakote for two weeks, and we've only been able to check the blood level once." I turned to Cindy. "What have you noticed that makes you think the Depakote might be helping?"

"Well, Jim was out of town for a few days last week, and so was my sister. I had the three kids twenty-four hours a day the whole time again. You know how keyed up I got the last time that happened."

In fact it had been a similar situation that had brought Cindy into treatment in the first place. About three weeks before our first meeting, Cindy had been with the three boys, six, five, and three years old, because of coinciding business trips taken by Jim and her sister. She had needed to call Jim and get him to fly back home because she was becoming more and more irritable with the children, snapping at them, slamming doors, starting to feel out of control.

The next week she had come to see me, and as we talked about her past history, it emerged that she had experienced episodes of depression after both her children were born, that she had had these "hyper" episodes about once a year since college, and that her mother had suffered from "mood swings" and alcoholism. A diagnosis of bipolar II or perhaps a "soft" bipolar disorder seemed likely, and we decided on a trial of a mood stabilizer.

"The kids just didn't get to me this time," Cindy continued. "First I thought they were being on their best behavior because of what had happened that last time, and maybe they were for an hour or so. But by evening I realized that they were really about as active as they usually are, and that there was something different about *me*. I wasn't as, you know, sensitive. Several times now I've noticed that I can handle things better."

"Not the other night," Jim chimed in. "I'm not noticing much difference."

"Well, maybe Jim's right," Cindy went on. "Maybe you could give me something for the times when I'm feeling really stressed? Some Valium or Xanax? I never used . . . I don't know what to call them—nerve pills? And I'm sure I wouldn't need them often."

"I don't think we should add more medication until we're sure you're getting the maximum benefit from the one you're on. And from what you're telling me, I think that's beginning to happen," I said. "The fact that you've never felt the need for tranquilizers before makes me think that the bipolar disorder explains all your symptoms and needs to be the focus of our attention. It's absolutely too early to expect the Depakote to have had its full effect. Also, your blood test indicates that we can safely raise the dose. Let's talk about this a bit more."

Cindy and Jim are very anxious for Cindy's symptoms to stop. Who can blame them? But to give up on a mood stabilizer after two weeks because it hasn't completely controlled every symptom is foolish. It's unlikely that another would work any faster—and it might not even work as well, in which case Cindy would be right back to square one after another couple of weeks.

Cindy's situation also serves to illustrate another principle of treatment: *remember the diagnosis.* If the three most important words in the real estate business are *location, location,* and *location,* then the three most important words in medicine are *diagnosis, diagnosis,* and *diagnosis.* Because we have so many effective medications, it can be tempting to consider prescribing one even though there isn't really a justification for it based on diagnosis. In psychiatry especially there was a tendency at one time to see medications as *symptomatic treatments*. This means picking a medication and making the decision to use it based on identification of *symptoms*, not underlying *diagnoses*. Cindy wants to try another medication for "stress"—that is, for feeling tense and irritable. But the symptoms of our working diagnosis, bipolar disorder, include periods of tension and irritability. If Cindy's poor stress tolerance is a symptom of her mood disorder, and she takes an anti-anxiety medication to cover it up rather than getting more intensive treatment of the mood disorder, she'll end up taking a medication she doesn't really need for a symptom that isn't going to get much better because the underlying problem, bipolar disorder, isn't being properly treated. Insomnia is a similar symptom, very commonly a symptom of the mood disorder but all too commonly treated with sleeping medications as if it were an isolated symptom.

Every once in a while I see a patient with bipolar disorder who has read a magazine article about attention deficit–hyperactivity disorder and requests medication for ADHD. Some of the symptoms of ADHD—like impulsivity, impatience, fast, disorganized thinking, and poor concentration—are, of course, also seen in bipolar patients. These are distressing symptoms that deserve attention, but they deserve the right kind of attention. If they are an expression of the mood changes of bipolar disorder, then medication for ADHD won't help. (In fact the medications used to treat ADHD, stimulants and antidepressants, can make things worse.)

Making a diagnosis is the process of identifying the one disease that can explain all the patient's symptoms. This is a variation of the scientific principle called Occam's razor. Named after William of Occam (or Ockham), the medieval theologian-philosopher who developed it, this principle states that the simplest explanation for a phenomenon is always preferable to a more complex one and is most likely to be correct. Obviously a patient may have two different disorders that require two different treatment approaches. But if all the patient's symptoms can be understood as expressions of *one* disorder, treating that one will likely alleviate all the symptoms.

I see this problem of multiple diagnoses and symptomatic treatments even more commonly in depressed patients. In depression, anxiety and insomnia can be thorny and uncomfortable expressions of the mood disorder—and physical symptoms can be as well, especially in the elderly. I have seen elderly patients taking antidepressant medications (often at an inadequate dose) who are also taking sleeping pills, tranquilizers, anti-inflammatory and pain medications for arthritis, stool softeners and laxatives for constipation, and sometimes some vitamins and tonics thrown in for good measure (perhaps because of complaints of "low energy"). All these problems are symptoms of depression, but sometimes it's hard to see the forest for the trees. Before you know it, the patient is taking a dozen or so different medications for all the different symptoms of depression, and the disease that underlies them all, a mood disorder, has been missed. It is an amazing experience to see all these symptoms that have not been helped by perhaps a dozen medications disappear after a week of ECT in an elderly patient.

This leads me to another principle: *ECT should not be a treatment of last resort for bipolar disorder.* ECT should be considered whenever symptoms are very severe, or when they are severe enough to interfere with work and family life and have gone on for an extended period of time. Some geriatric psychiatrists are recommending ECT as the *first-line treatment* for serious mood-disorder symptoms in the elderly. If the patient is having symptoms day after day, has been on medical leave from work for weeks, and is still not getting relief from his or her medication, it's time to seriously consider ECT. When symptoms are disabling, ECT should probably be considered after the failure of the first medication, not after the failure of the second or third or fourth.

Finally, I can't stress enough that *every bipolar patient needs psychotherapy* at one point or another. Several weeks or months of counseling is absolutely essential after the diagnosis and initiation of treatment for bipolar disorder. Just as a person with diabetes needs to follow dietary recommendations to get the best control of his or her glucose levels, and a hip-fracture patient needs physical therapy for optimal functioning, persons with bipolar disorder need psychotherapy at times to have the best possible control of their mood symptoms.

PART III

VARIATIONS, CAUSES, AND CONNECTIONS

In this group of chapters we'll explore several variations on the theme of bipolar disorder. We'll look first at how the course and symptoms of the illness can differ in children and adolescents and then consider the differences in symptoms between men and women (with special attention to premenstrual mood symptoms, the challenge of postpartum mood disorders, and the dilemmas faced by women with the illness during the childbearing years).

In chapter 15 we'll look at the complicated relationships between bipolar disorder and substance abuse. Individuals with bipolar disorder seem to be especially vulnerable to substance-abuse disorders, so much so that it's reasonable to think of chemical dependency as a complication of the illness. The symptoms of substance abuse and bipolar disorder can become so intertwined that it is impossible to figure out which is which. In this chapter we'll look for a way out of this confusion and discuss the treatment approaches that work for individuals who have bipolar disorder complicated by chemical dependency. It's extremely important to deal with this problem head on, because research shows that alcoholism and drug abuse are often *fatal* complications of this illness.

In chapter 16 we'll learn about treating mood disorders with light, and about the intricate relationships between mood and the body's biological clock. We ignore what this clock tells us at our peril, because our sleep-wake cycle may help regulate our mood state. This is one aspect of mood regulation that we are beginning to understand in greater and greater detail. Persons with mood disorder owe it to themselves to learn as much as they can about these new findings.

In the last several chapters in this part of the book, we'll go from one extreme to the other as far as causes and connections are concerned, looking first at some very concrete scientific issues and then at some very abstract, almost philosophical ones. In chapter 17 we'll explore an area of intense interest to bipolar patients and their family members: the genetics of bipolar disorder. Chapter 18 looks at more bipolar biology: how mood disorders can be caused by medical illnesses, some of the ways we are actually picturing bipolar disorder in the functioning brain, and, finally, the possible connections between bipolar disorder and viruses.

Then, after we've finished talking about DNA molecules and chromosomes and brain chemicals, we'll leave the laboratory and go into the artist's studio, to examine some of the intriguing connections between this terrible illness and artistic genius and creativity.

CHAPTER 13

Bipolar Disorder in Children and Adolescents

FOR MANY YEARS BIPOLAR DISORDER WAS THOUGHT TO BE EXTREMELY rare in young people, even though research data on adults indicated that the first appearance of the symptoms of bipolar disorder usually occurs before the age of twenty. (Emil Kraepelin found that the highest number of "first attacks" of manic-depressive illness occurred between the ages of fifteen and twenty.) Perhaps because of a reluctance to diagnose children with an illness known to be a lifelong problem and to prescribe children the powerful medications used to treat its symptoms, bipolar disorder in young children received little attention from researchers until quite recently. This means that the treatment of children and adolescents with bipolar symptoms has consisted mostly of improvised variations on adult treatments. More research has shown, however, that bipolar disorder in children and adolescents may not be the same as bipolar disorder in adults. Therefore, different treatment approaches may be necessary in younger patients.

Although research on bipolar disorder is beginning to show that it is probably not as rare in children as was once thought, the kind of large sampling study it would take to determine the prevalence of bipolar disorder in children hasn't yet been undertaken. But the studies that are available indicate that very young children can have bipolar symptoms. In one study that looked at bipolar symptoms in the pediatric (under eighteen) age range, nearly a third of the patients were younger than twelve, and the average age of onset for these young bipolar patients was eight and a half.[1] This same research is also shedding light on why psychiatrists used to think pediatric bipolar disorder was a rare diagnosis: bipolar disorder in children doesn't look the same as bipolar

TABLE 13-1 Comparison of Adult and Pediatric Bipolar Disorder

	Pediatric	Adult
Initial episode:	Major depression	Mania
Episode type:	Rapid cycling, mixed	Discrete episodes
Duration:	Chronic, continuous	Weeks
Functioning between episodes:	Poor (continuous cycling)	Improved

disorder in adults. If you look for adult symptom patterns in young children, you won't find them very often.

It appears that when bipolar disorder occurs in young children (before puberty), it is a more severe form of the illness. Perhaps this is because children who develop symptoms of bipolar disorder at so young an age seem to have a heavier genetic "loading" for mood disorders than do people with older-adolescent- and adult-onset bipolar disorder. Bipolar children often have more individuals with mood disorders in their families than adult-diagnosis bipolar patients; many of these children have individuals with mood disorders on both sides of the family.[2] Another difference between childhood- and adult-onset bipolar disorder is that rather than mania or hypomania, a major depression is frequently the first sign of the disorder in children. Several studies indicate that 20 to 30 percent of young people with major depressions go on to develop manic symptoms later in life.[3]

But the most striking difference between childhood-onset and later-onset bipolar disorder is the course of the illness. Pediatric bipolar disorder is a much more continuous illness than adult bipolar disorder. In most adults the illness usually appears in discrete episodes of depression or mania, and the symptoms go into remission for months or years at a time. Children, on the other hand, often have long periods of continuous rapid cycling. These children sometimes cycle between depression and mania several times a day, having a laughing fit one moment and talking about wanting to shoot themselves the next.[4] One study of bipolar disorder in the pediatric age range described bipolar children who had over a hundred mini-manias in a year, mood episodes that lasted only a day or two. In this study, none of the research subjects under the age of nine had a single mood episode lasting two weeks or more as his or her only episode. In these children a complex pattern of frequent, short episodes was the rule, not the exception.[5]

Symptoms of Pediatric Bipolar Disorder

Depression is comparatively easy to spot in children: the weepy, listless, and lethargic child is quickly recognized as a sick child. But how do you distinguish hypomanic or manic behavior in a child from the boisterousness and high energy of normal children? An even more difficult task is to differentiate manic symptoms from the hyperactivity and "can't sit still" picture of attention deficit–hyperactivity disorder (ADHD).

The differentiation is possible if close attention is paid to changes in mood. Children with ADHD are hyperactive but don't have the expansive, grandiose mood of mania. The child with ADHD may disrupt a classroom with clowning around and restlessness, but a manic child may tell the teacher that the lessons are being taught incorrectly and try to take over the class. The manic child caught taking things that belong to someone else may say that it's wrong for other people to steal but not for him or her. The manic child may be convinced that he or she is destined for a brilliant career as a doctor or lawyer despite failing nearly every subject in school. The child may believe that he or she is on the verge of becoming a rock star despite being unable to play a musical instrument.

Normal children, of course, will fantasize in similar ways about their future, but they will be able to separate their fantasies from reality and will apply themselves to school work and follow the rules at home. Manic children, on the other hand, convinced of the reality of their grandiose ideas, state and act on the belief that the usual rules and requirements don't apply to them.

Manic children jump from topic to topic in their speech patterns, are difficult to interrupt, and complain that their thoughts are moving too fast. Hypersexuality is a symptom in older children, who may become sexually promiscuous or masturbate excessively; they may suddenly start using sexual profanity or express the belief that a teacher or famous person is in love with them. Spending sprees may take the form of ordering items over the phone using 1-800 and 1-900 numbers.

Very young children may have manic exaggerations of the normal magical thinking of childhood but will act on this thinking instead of using it as a basis for play. Normal children may imagine that they can fly and may run through the back yard "flapping" their arms like the wings of a bird or making airplane noises. Manic children under the influence of the delusion that they've become an angel or a superhero may jump out of a window or off the roof of a house. The symptoms of bipolar disorder in children can be every bit as deadly as they are in adults.

Bipolar Disorder and ADHD

As more research has been done on bipolar disorder in children and adolescents, it has become clear that some young people who are "hyperactive" do not have attention deficit–hyperactivity disorder but instead have bipolar disorder. But this research also points to some relationships between the two diagnoses, relationships that at this point are still poorly understood.

It is possible to differentiate between the symptoms of ADHD and those of childhood bipolar disorder in many children, but some children seem to have both disorders simultaneously. In one study of children who had already been diagnosed with ADHD, 11 percent were also found to meet diagnostic criteria for bipolar disorder—that is, they seemed to have both disorders. When this group was reevaluated four years later, another 15 percent of the ADHD children met diagnostic criteria for bipolar disorder. This suggests that in some children, at least, ADHD symptoms may in fact be early signs of bipolar disorder. The ADHD children who eventually developed bipolar symptoms had more severe symptoms and more disturbed behaviors.[6]

Most children with ADHD gradually grow out of it. Their ability to concentrate improves, and their impulsivity and hyperactivity gradually diminish as they grow into adolescence and adulthood. Occasionally some of the symptoms persist into adulthood, but when they do, the adults have attention and concentration problems, not problems with mood regulation. Bipolar disorder, on the other hand, usually accelerates as the individual ages. So how do we understand the children whose ADHD seems to develop into bipolar disorder? Did they really have ADHD symptoms in the first place, or does very-early-onset bipolar disorder mimic ADHD in its early stages? And what do we make of the children who seem to have both illnesses simultaneously? Are ADHD and pediatric bipolar disorder two separate illnesses that share similar symptom pictures but have different causes? Can ADHD develop into bipolar disorder? If so, how? The answers to these questions are not yet known, and the nature of the connection between ADHD and pediatric bipolar disorder is unclear. It has been suggested that the link may be genetic.[7] Perhaps these are two separate illnesses that happen to be inherited together frequently because the genes that cause them are close to one another on the chromosome and are thus usually inherited together. The only thing really sure about this mysterious connection is that much research in the area remains to be done.

Treatment and Prognosis

The treatment of pediatric bipolar disorder is still evolving. As you might expect, most of our treatment experience has been with lithium. Several studies indicate that lithium is effective in children, but there is also some evidence that it is not as effective in children as in adults. If complicated rapid-cycling bipolar disorder is indeed the rule in early-onset bipolar disorder, then lithium resistance should not be a big surprise: similar types of bipolar symptoms seem relatively lithium-resistant in adults, too. Pediatric lithium doses are, of course, lower than adult doses, but the effective therapeutic range for lithium in the bloodstream when it does work seems to be about the same in children as in adults. (Remember that the therapeutic range in the bloodstream is a measure of lithium concentration. Because children have a smaller total blood volume than adults, a lower dose of lithium for a child will result in the same concentration in the bloodstream.) Getting regular blood tests done is, of course, more challenging with children than with adults, but given the toxicity of lithium, blood levels are if anything even more important in children. Several studies have been done using methods that avoid the needles, taking lithium levels from saliva rather than from blood, but the results have been disappointing, and so for now these little patients must, unfortunately, have blood tests.

The efficacy in children of other adult treatments for bipolar disorder—anticonvulsants, antipsychotic medications, and so forth—has been reported on here and there, but not enough research has been done to provide definitive recommendations regarding first-line treatment for children. Improvisation is, unfortunately, still necessary to some extent. Much work remains to be done to determine the optimum treatment approach for childhood bipolar disorder.[8]

How is normal psychological development in children affected by bipolar disorder? Relationships with family members are often strained for these patients, as are relationships with peers. Their educational development inevitably suffers as well. Clearly, attention to the psychological needs and the special educational requirements of these children is vitally important to minimize the effects of the illness on their psychological development. Thus, perhaps even more than in adults, counseling and therapy must be a high priority when developing treatment plans for children with bipolar disorder.

Does earlier onset of bipolar symptoms predict a stormier course of illness later on? As noted previously, children frequently have continuous rapid cycling and mixed symptoms. Does the illness take on the more usual adult pattern of discrete episodes as these children age? If so, are the episodes more frequent than in persons with later-onset illness? The jury is still out on this question, and research results are lacking. But at least one small study shows that bipolar disorder in young persons can indeed be a difficult illness to manage. In this study, fifty-four adolescents who were admitted to a university hospital with a diagnosis of bipolar I disorder were followed for five years.[9] Of these youngsters, nearly half had a relapse, and about half of these had two or more episodes during the five years of the study. This study was done on patients who needed to be admitted to the hospital, and so it is biased toward looking at sicker patients. This type of research problem is called *ascertainment bias:* the results of the study may be skewed because of the method used to gather patients for the study. In this case, since patients who were not ill enough to need hospitalization would not have made it into the study, the study group may not be representative of all pediatric bipolar I patients. Nevertheless, these results would seem to indicate that at least some of these young patients are especially prone to relapse and so need careful monitoring.

But as to the longer course of bipolar disorder that begins in childhood, there is practically no information. Is the course of illness different at age thirty or forty depending on whether it started at the age of ten or at twenty? There are no definitive answers to this sort of question for now.

Several tasks lie ahead for those researching bipolar disorder in children. First will be to improve upon the diagnostic process and find out how to better separate bipolar (especially manic) symptoms from other similar diagnostic pictures—especially attention deficit–hyperactivity disorder. Clarifying the relationship between bipolar disorder and ADHD will be a very instructive area of research for other reasons as well and will surely lead to better understanding of and treatments for both disorders. More research to determine which of the available treatments for bipolar disorder work best for children and adolescents is also needed, as are long-term follow-up studies to see if pediatric-onset bipolar disorder looks different from late-adolescent-onset bipolar disorder as the patient grows to adulthood.

CHAPTER 14

Women with Bipolar Disorder: Special Considerations

ALTHOUGH WOMEN ARE NO MORE LIKELY THAN MEN TO SUFFER FROM bipolar disorder, the hormonal changes that accompany menstruation and pregnancy affect the course of bipolar disorder in women and deserve special attention, as do some patterns of symptoms more often experienced by women than men with bipolar disorder. Finally, medication use during pregnancy and while breast-feeding requires careful consideration.

Premenstrual Syndromes

There has been intense interest for many years in the mood symptoms that many women experience for several days before the monthly onset of menstruation. The *DSM IV* contains a description of *premenstrual dysphoric disorder,* with diagnostic criteria that include depressed mood, change in energy level and appetite, and physical symptoms like bloating and breast tenderness. (Premenstrual dysphoric disorder is not in the main part of the *DSM* but rather in an appendix called "Criteria Sets and Axes Provided for Further Study." This means that the diagnosis is not well enough understood and characterized for the experts to agree on what should constitute diagnostic criteria.) The most common designation for mood symptoms that cycle with menstruation continues to be *premenstrual syndrome,* or *PMS.* Is PMS a separate disorder, or is it an "ordinary" mood disorder whose symptoms simply fluctuate with the hormonal changes of the menstrual cycle? This is the big unanswered question about PMS, and one of the reasons why PMS is not in the *DSM* as an "official" diagnosis. Investigations into things like hormone levels in patients with PMS have not, for the most part, found anything abnormal. Moreover, the best relief from the symptoms of PMS seems to come from the usual treatments for mood disorders, rather than hormonal treatments. Another confusing factor in the study of PMS is the finding that many, perhaps even most, women experience some unpleasant physical and psychological symptoms for a few days prior to the onset of menstrual flow. Finding a group of women with "PMS" whose symptoms can be clearly distinguished from those of women with "normal" premenstrual symptoms and whose timing and profile of symptoms clearly separate them from women with other mood disorders is a clinical research challenge still unmet.

The situation with bipolar disorder is just as murky: some studies indicate that the timing of bipolar symptoms relates to the menstrual cycle, and others have not found any such relationship. In a study wherein women with bipolar disorder were given questionnaires asking about premenstrual symptoms, 60 percent reported a worsening of symptoms premenstrually. But since this is a *retrospective* study—patients were asked to remember something that had happened in the past—the results are highly questionable. Retrospective studies, especially questionnaire studies, are handicapped by the known tendency of people to connect their symptoms to events in their past and try to make sense of them in this way; people tend to overstate their symptoms in questionnaires and make connections where there aren't any. In another study of bipolar disorder and the menstrual cycle, the research subjects rated their moods every day, making it a *prospective* study—usually considered to be a better research technique. In this study *no association* between mood symptoms and menstrual cycles was found in a group of women with rapid-cycling bipolar disorder. But in a study looking at hospitalization, it was found that women with bipolar disorder were more likely to be hospitalized during the premenstrual and menstrual phases of the menstrual cycle than at other times.[1]

So the relationship between bipolar symptoms and the menstrual cycle is still unclear. There may be a group of women with bipolar disorder who are at higher risk for developing symptoms premenstrually, but how this should affect their treatment is unknown.

I can't leave behind the subject of premenstrual mood symptoms without mentioning an intriguing study published in the *American Journal of Psychiatry* in 1997.[2] The researchers had noticed that there is a significant overlap between PMS symptoms and the symptoms of seasonal affective disorder (SAD). In both syndromes depressed mood is accompanied by low energy, a tendency to sleep too much rather than too little, and an increase in appetite with carbohydrate craving. (We'll go into the details of the symptoms of SAD in chapter 16.) When the researchers asked patients referred to a PMS clinic if their PMS was worse during the winter, about two-thirds said that it was. Thirty-eight percent of the original group met diagnostic criteria for full-blown seasonal affective disorder. These women, then, had a mood disorder that cycled in at least *two* ways: with the monthly menstrual cycle, and with the twelve-month cycle of the seasons. This study shows us once more that there are intricate and complex relationships between mood and bodily rhythms and cycles, and that mood disorders are affected by many different factors in ways we are only beginning to understand.

Symptom Differences in Women

Of the various differences between the genders in the course of illness and symptoms of bipolar disorder, the greater incidence of rapid cycling in women is the best documented. A review article on bipolar disorder in women looked at ten studies involving several hundred persons with rapid-cycling bipolar disorder and found that 74 percent of the rapid-cycling patients were female.[3] Thus, the ratio of women to men with rapid-cycling disorder is 3:1.

Several reasons have been proposed for this difference. Since thyroid problems have been associated with rapid cycling in bipolar disorder, and since women are more likely than men to have certain types of thyroid problems, it was thought that a higher incidence of thyroid disease among women might explain the difference. But when women with rapid-cycling bipolar disorder were tested for thyroid problems, no greater incidence of thyroid disease was found. Theories implicating female hormones have also been suggested, but so far they are mostly speculative, and no research data exist clearly proving that hormonal differences between men and women explain this difference.

Another intriguing idea about the increased incidence of rapid-cycling bipolar disorder in women is related to the finding that women with bipolar disorder have a slightly greater ratio of depressive to manic episodes than men have. Several studies have found that women with bipolar disorder tend to have more episodes of depression during the course of their illness than men have.[4] This being the case, it may be that women with bipolar disorder are more likely to be treated with antidepressants that can cause them to enter a rapid-cycling phase of the disorder. The types of clinical studies that would prove this theory have yet to be carried out.

The finding that women with bipolar disorder have more depressive episodes than their male counterparts seems to fit with the finding that women are more likely than men to suffer from nonbipolar depression. No one understands this greater tendency of women to suffer from depressive illnesses. As I noted above, research on the levels of the female reproductive hormones in depressed women has generally been unrevealing.

It is now known that there are many differences in brain organization between women and men, differences that have little to do with sex and reproduction. Psychological testing profiles indicate that women are superior to men in their performance on certain tests of language and memory, and men perform better on certain specialized tests of three-dimensional visualization. It is thought that there are subtle differences in the way the brains of men and women are "wired" during prenatal development, probably under the influence of hormones in the womb, especially testosterone. The differences between men and women in the incidence and symptom profile of mood disorders may be due to these differences in "wiring." Explaining the significantly higher incidence of serious depression, including bipolar depression, in women is perhaps the most important unanswered question before us in the field of women's mental health.

Postpartum Mood Disorders and Family Planning

Emil Kraepelin noticed that women often had episodes of mania after giving birth, and for many years the term *postpartum psychosis* was a familiar one in medicine. With the reawakening of interest in careful diagnosis in psychiatry, however, it has become clear that most of these episodes of "psychosis" are episodes of bipolar disorder. Many clinical studies indicate that women with bipolar disorder are at very high risk for an episode of illness in the period after giving birth. One review article on bipolar disorder in women put it this way: "There is no other time in the life of a male or female bipolar patient when the risk of an episode is higher than it is for a female bipolar patient in the post-partum period."[5] One can speculate on the reasons for this: the emotional and physical stress of labor and delivery with the inevitable sleep deprivation, periods of physical pain, and dramatic changes in the levels of reproductive and stress hormones that attend childbirth. But the exact reasons for this very striking finding remain unknown.

Women with bipolar disorder who want to have a child are thus faced with a challenging dilemma. On the one hand, physicians usually recommend that a woman not take any medications during pregnancy, in order to protect the unborn child from prenatal exposure to pharmaceuticals. On the other hand, it is clear that a woman with bipolar disorder is at high risk for relapse after giving birth and perhaps needs medication late in her pregnancy more than at any other time in her life. Another problem is that the most commonly used mood-stabilizing medications—lithium, valproate, and carbamazepine—all have been associated with birth defects.

There are no easy solutions to these problems, but a few facts suggest some ways out. Most embryonic development has been completed by the final months of pregnancy, and lithium may be safer during pregnancy than originally thought. Current recommendations include avoiding most medications, especially the ones most closely linked to birth defects, during the early months of pregnancy and restarting treatment as soon as possible after delivery, possibly even in the latter stages of pregnancy.

But this much is very clear: simply stopping all medications while trying to get pregnant and for the duration of the pregnancy in order to eliminate all risk to the fetus is *very* risky for the mother. Some women will, of course, be willing to take this risk, and there are many arguments to support this approach. On the other hand, the first weeks and months—and some say the first few moments—of mother-child contact are very important for mother-child bonding, and this process may be disrupted if the mother is depressed or hospitalized with bipolar symptoms.

Many women with bipolar disorder have healthy babies and remain well in the weeks and months following delivery. Careful planning, conscientious symptom monitoring, and timely resumption of treatment will probably increase the chances of this happening. The woman with bipolar disorder owes it to herself and to her child to think and plan carefully about pregnancy. She should find an obstetrician and a psychiatrist who will support her decision to become pregnant and work closely with her and with each other toward the healthiest possible outcome for both mother and baby.

Is it safe to breast-feed while taking medication? Many medications are secreted in breast milk, but there is little research about the effects of these medications on infants. Although the Food and Drug Administration has not approved any psychiatric medication for use during breast-feeding, a few clinics provide careful monitoring for infant exposure to pharmaceuticals by testing breast milk and the baby's blood and urine, thus making it possible for some of their patients to breast-feed more safely while taking medications.[6]

Alcoholism and Drug Abuse

OF ALL THE STATISTICS ASSOCIATED WITH BIPOLAR DISORDER, HERE is one of the most significant and most disturbing: according to one very important study, more than 60 percent of persons with bipolar disorder also suffer from alcoholism or drug-abuse problems.[1]

Does having bipolar disorder make individuals more likely to use and abuse drugs and alcohol? Can alcoholism or drug abuse trigger the development of bipolar disorder in someone who is genetically vulnerable? Do bipolar disorder and substance-abuse disorders have a common biochemical or genetic cause? There is evidence to support an answer of yes to all of these questions.

Bipolar Binges

Perhaps the easiest-to-understand model for the observed link between bipolar disorder and alcoholism and drug abuse is the idea that the mood changes of bipolar disorder propel people into situations they would otherwise be able to avoid and cause them to do things they otherwise wouldn't do.

Brad was a forty-two-year-old writer. He had a day job as a copywriter for a small advertising firm, but his creative juices really started flowing late at night when he worked on his "stories." In college Brad had won a writing contest and had seen his very first attempt at writing a short story published in a prestigious national publication. Since then he had published one or two stories a year, sometimes in little literary journals that paid him practically nothing, once in *Atlantic Monthly,* most often in something in between.

I first met Brad when he was starting to get treatment for alcoholism at the substance-abuse treatment facility affiliated with the hospital where I worked. A psychiatric consultation had been requested because Brad had told the staff he had been troubled by depression and thought it made his drinking problems worse.

"I know what you're thinking: another alcoholic writer. But I'm not."

"Slow down, Brad," I said. "I didn't even know you were a writer until you told me just now." He was a serious and intense man with dark, deep-set eyes. I had to admit he looked the part of the troubled writer. "But I'm interested in hearing your ideas about your drinking problem."

"Sorry, I shouldn't jump to conclusions. But people always think of writers as alcoholics. You know, Hemingway, Tennessee Williams, sitting at their typewriters with a glass of Scotch. Well, I don't drink when I write, I drink when I can't write."

This was beginning to sound interesting. "What do you mean?" I asked.

Brad drank when he couldn't write because it made him feel better. And it gradually became clear to me that when he couldn't write, it was because he was depressed. "My mind just goes blank for days at a time. I get behind at work, I sleep too much, and I don't even bother turning the computer on at home. I can get the car-wax and potato-chip commercials written at work, but I couldn't be really creative if my life depended on it. This 'what's the use?' feeling comes over me, and I find myself bringing home a fifth of vodka two or three times a week and just sipping the nights away."

"Have you ever used any other drugs? Marijuana? Cocaine?" I asked.

"Oh, yes," Brad said with a deep sigh. "About three years ago I drained my bank account over a summer—blew it all on cocaine. If I hadn't ended up in the hospital, I might never have stopped."

"What happened?"

"Well, this is really embarrassing. I don't know what got into me, but I got this inspiration to try writing for TV. I had never tried scriptwriting before, but I was sure I could do it. I got an idea for a script about a guy who falls in love with a woman with a cocaine problem. I thought I needed to do some research—you know, where you go to buy the stuff, what those areas of town are like, the people involved."

"Maybe you should have tried the library first."

Brad turned, looking at me intently. At first I thought I had offended him with my little attempt at humor. But I hadn't. "That's just it," he said. "That what I usually *would* have done." He looked away again. "I'm not a particularly brave person, and certainly not a fool. But I was . . . I don't know quite how to put it . . . uninhibited, confident. I found myself walking down streets at midnight that I would have been nervous walking down in broad daylight. I bought the stuff and had no qualms about using it. And I was hooked in no time at all. I would get off work, go home, and write until it got dark. Then I'd make a run for the cocaine, kind of cruise around for a while, then come home and snort it. I'd get back to the writing and go at it until the sun came up."

"When did you sleep?" I asked.

"I didn't, not for days at a time. I didn't need to. I felt energized all the time."

"All the time?"

"Yes, I think cocaine must affect me differently than it does most people. I was feeling high even hours and hours after I had used. Once the high lasted three days."

This was sounding like more than just a drug and alcohol problem. People don't feel high from cocaine for three days. Something else had energized Brad that summer. His mood and behavioral changes had all the hallmarks of hypomania.

"So how did you end up in the hospital?"

"One morning my heart started beating real fast and my chest started to hurt. I left the office and got myself to the emergency room. They wanted to admit me right away, but I wouldn't let them."

"Why not?"

"It didn't seem necessary to me. I thought my heart was fine; I just wanted something for the pain. I know that sounds crazy now, but I think I *was* a little crazy by then. I don't remember much about what happened next, but they told me I started shouting and fighting. All I know is I got two shots in the butt and didn't wake up until eleven hours later."

Fortunately Brad's heart *was* fine, but he was discharged with a prescription for Risperdal to take for a few days for what was called a "cocaine-induced psychosis." His sleep patterns and energy level got back to normal.

"It's funny," he added, "I haven't had even the slightest temptation to use cocaine again. I didn't drink either for the whole next year. But then I found myself slipping into the pit again, and I didn't have the energy to say no anymore. But this time I knew I needed help. I think memories of that cocaine summer made me realize that the drinking might lead to something else again if I didn't get some serious treatment. That's why I checked in here."

I couldn't help asking one more question before telling Brad I thought he probably had bipolar disorder: "Did you finish the script?"

"Yes, I did. It turned out great. I've sent it to a producer, and she's interested. You know, I might even make back the money I spent on my, uh . . . research."

Not all stories like Brad's have such a happy ending. Some persons with bipolar disorder can indeed pull out of substance abuse when their mood episodes come to an end, either spontaneously or with treatment, but for others the substance-abuse problem takes on a life of its own. In the worst-case scenario, the mood disorder and the substance-abuse disorder start feeding on each other, and a vicious cycle of mood symptoms, increased substance abuse, and even more severe mood fluctuations takes over until it's impossible to separate one problem from the other.

Psychiatrists used to talk a great deal about "self-medication" in discussing the relationship between bipolar disorder and substance abuse. The idea was that bipolar patients sometimes started down the road to a full-blown substance-abuse problem by attempting to "treat" their mood symptoms with alcohol or drugs of abuse. Although this certainly occurs in some patients, it doesn't seem to be the most common scenario. Although some patients, like Brad, find themselves drinking while depressed because it deadens the psychic pain of depression, bipolar patients seem at greater risk for alcohol and drug abuse when they are hypomanic or manic. Brad's cocaine binge is actually the more typical story. The "self-medication" hypothesis might predict that bipolar patients would use stimulants like cocaine to alleviate their depressions. But studies show that, like Brad, bipolar patients are more likely to use cocaine—and to a lesser extent alcohol—to intensify and prolong their hypomanic and manic states.[2]

The link between mania and cocaine abuse has convinced many researchers that it is manic disinhibition and loss of judgment rather than a tendency to "self-medicate" that puts bipolar patients at such high risk for substance abuse.

Effect, Cause, or Association?

Another possible relationship between bipolar disorder and substance abuse works in the other direction—that is, alcohol and drug abuse may bring on episodes of abnormal mood in bipolar-disorder patients, perhaps by triggering episodes in persons who are vulnerable to the disorder because of genetic factors. Several studies have shown that bipolar patients who have a substance-abuse disorder have a stormier course to their mood disorder than patients who do not abuse alcohol or drugs. "Dual-diagnosis" patients, on average, first develop symptoms of their bipolar disorder at a younger age, and in some studies they have been shown to have more frequent hospitalizations. This has been interpreted to indicate that substance abuse may worsen the course of bipolar disorder, perhaps because of some direct effect on the brain of repeated use of drugs and alcohol.[3]

Finally, it may be that, like bipolar disorder, a vulnerability to addiction has a strong genetic component, and the two problems tend to occur together simply because the genes for both are located close to one another on the chromosomes and tend to be inherited together. I, for one, have seen too many patients like Brad—patients whose bipolar-disorder symptoms and substance abuse seem to trigger and reinforce each other—to believe that these so often tightly intertwined problems are randomly associated.

Use or Abuse?

At what point does substance use become "abuse"? It would be easy for me to launch into a long and complex discussion of diagnostic criteria for substance abuse and chemical dependency, but that probably wouldn't be very helpful. I think the issue is quite clear for individuals with a mood disorder: with the possible exception of occasional alcohol use, I advise persons with a mood disorder to *scrupulously avoid any and all intoxicating substances in any quantity whatsoever.*

All abused substances appear to work by stimulating "reward" centers in the brain. You have probably heard that laboratory animals will push a lever that delivers an electrical stimulus to certain brain regions rather than another one that delivers food to their cage, and will continue doing so until they're practically dead from hunger. When a similar lever device is used to deliver an intravenous dose of alcohol or another drug to laboratory animals, the substances that animals will willingly and persistently self-administer in this way are almost exactly the same ones that humans use to get intoxicated: narcotics, cocaine, and certain stimulants and tranquilizers. These are the same substances that humans abuse and become addicted to. Some drugs, like cocaine, affect these centers quickly and powerfully; others, like marijuana, work more slowly, but they all work the same way: by disrupting the normal operation of the brain's "feel-good" circuitry.

Now, you don't need to be a psychiatrist to realize that persons with bipolar disorder already have enough problems with the "feel-good" circuits of the brain, and that mucking things up further with "recreational" drugs is a *very* bad idea. There is some evidence to suggest that intoxicating substances actively interfere with the therapeutic effects of the medications used to treat mood disorders. It seems to me that *any* use of intoxicating substances by persons with bipolar disorder is unhealthy and extremely risky and for those reasons amounts to substance abuse.

The question that usually comes next is, Can't I even have an occasional glass of wine with dinner? Although I'm hard-pressed to forbid my patients ever to drink, it's clear that when it comes to alcohol, less is better. Given the known high risk of bipolar patients for serious substance-abuse problems, the best course is probably no alcohol at all.

A Deadly Combination

There is one well-established research finding that is much more significant than all the speculation about the nature of the association between bipolar disorder and substance abuse and even more disturbing than the extremely high rate of substance abuse among people with bipolar disorder. This is the finding that persons who have mood disorders and also abuse alcohol or drugs have a greatly increased risk of completed suicide. Severe depression complicated by alcoholism or drug abuse has been found to be one of the most frequent diagnostic pictures in study after study of the psychiatric diagnoses of suicide victims. In a 1993 study attempting to make psychiatric diagnoses on suicide victims, clinicians reviewed the medical records and interviewed the relatives of almost fourteen hundred persons who had committed suicide. This study, which found that most of the suicide victims had suffered from a mood disorder, also found that *nearly half* (48 percent) had suffered from alcoholism or drug abuse.[4]

Another point to emphasize here is that when bipolar disorder and a

TABLE 15-1 Signs of Alcoholism

Many medical and professional organizations endorse the CAGE questionnaire to identify problem drinking:

1. Have you ever felt you should **C**ut down on your drinking?
2. Have people **A**nnoyed you by criticizing your drinking?
3. Have you ever felt bad or **G**uilty about your drinking?
4. Have you ever had a drink first thing in the morning to steady your nerves or get rid of a hangover (an **E**ye opener)?

One *yes* suggests a possible alcohol problem. More than one *yes* means that an alcohol problem is highly likely.

Source: National Institute on Alcohol Abuse and Alcoholism, *Alcoholism: Getting the Facts,* 1996.

substance-abuse problem coexist, they *both* need treatment. Getting proper treatment for the mood disorder will certainly make the substance-abuse problem easier to treat, but it cannot be assumed that a substance-abuse problem will simply go away when a coexisting mood disorder is treated. An active substance-abuse problem will in fact make the mood disorder difficult to diagnose, let alone treat.

Psychiatrists and other mental-health professionals are well versed in the available treatment resources in their community for chemical-dependency problems. But perhaps more than most other types of mental-health problems, the treatment of alcohol- and drug-abuse problems requires a wide range of specialized services and support groups. Mental-health professionals will usually refer a patient to a chemical-dependency center or organization for evaluation and treatment of a chemical dependency. Treatment options might include in-patient rehabilitation, out-patient treatment, or a new type of treatment program wherein patients spend the day at the program and return home at night. There are even evening programs that allow people to return to work during the day.

The first step is admitting that there might be a problem. This is often the most difficult step. When in doubt, talking about these concerns with the psychiatrist or therapist is not just important, it can be literally lifesaving.

CHAPTER 16

Seasonal Affective Disorder and Chronobiology

CHRONOBIOLOGY (FROM *KHRONOS,* THE GREEK WORD FOR "TIME") IS the science of bodily rhythms and biological clocks. Nearly every organism on the planet lives in rhythm with the astronomical cycles of the earth, sun, and moon. The activities of animals and the growth cycles of plants harmonize with the daily rising and setting of the sun, the monthly ebb and flow of ocean tides, the annual cycle of the changing seasons.

Ancient peoples erected immense astronomical calculators and observatories like Stonehenge in England and the monuments at Carnac in France, where rows of more than a thousand stones stretch across the countryside. At these sacred places and at others, like the pyramids of the Mayans and Incas, ancient astronomers determined the dates and times of solstices, equinoxes, and eclipses. In festivals like the Roman Saturnalia our forebears celebrated the lengthening of the daylight hours that heralds the arrival of spring and the return of the sun. Our modern midwinter holidays, Christmas and Hanukkah, recall these sentiments with traditions centered around candles, lights, and greenery.

Once we humans learned how to predict eclipses, we were no longer terrified by them. As we learned how to extend the daylight hours with fire and gaslight and electricity, we depended less on the cycles of the sun to structure our activities and felt more in control of time. We learned to warm ourselves in winter and cool ourselves in summer. The changes of seasons were still lovely to watch and interesting in the way they affected the plants and animals around us, but they didn't really affect us very much anymore—or so we thought.

But the changes of the seasons certainly *do* affect other creatures: the migration of birds, salmon, and whales, Arctic rabbits that change color in winter, the astonishing changes in plant life that occur from fall to winter to spring, and, of course, those hibernating bears. But humans have evolved beyond all that, haven't we? Our cycles of activity, like our sleeping at night and being awake during the day, are just conventions set by our culture rather than expressions of our biology. We humans have severed our connections with the rhythms of the celestial bodies. Haven't we?

That's what many of us thought—until 1982, when a paper by researchers from the National Institutes of Mental Health appeared in the *American Journal of Psychiatry*.[1] This paper, called "Bright Artificial Light Treatment of a Manic-Depressive Patient with a Seasonal Mood Cycle," described a patient with bipolar disorder whose symptoms occurred in a pattern related to the seasons: depression in winter and mood elevation during the summer.

Seasonal patterns in bipolar disorder had been described previously by a number of astute clinicians, including (as you might expect) Emil Kraepelin, who observed, "Repeatedly in these cases, I saw moodiness set in in autumn and pass over in spring 'when the sap shoots in the trees,' to excitement."[2] But there had been little organized research activity into the relationship between mood and the seasons. Then in the late 1970s a group of researchers were drawn together at NIMH by a mutual interest in seasonal mood changes, and they started to look at these relationships. One of them, Norman Rosenthal, had noticed his own seasonal shifts of mood for a number of years in his native South Africa, and had seen these mood swings worsen when his psychiatric training brought him to New York—a city located much farther from the equator than his native Johannesburg had been. In New York the summer days are much longer and the winter days much shorter than in South Africa. Rosenthal recalled his first autumn in New York this way:

> Daylight-saving time was over and the clocks were put back an hour.
> I left that first Monday after the time change and found the world in
> darkness. A cold wind blowing off the Hudson River filled me with
> foreboding. Winter came. My energy declined, and I wondered how
> I could have undertaken so many tasks the previous summer. Had
> I been crazy? Now there seemed to be no alternative but to hang in and
> try to keep everything afloat . . . Finally, spring arrived. My energy level
> surged again, and I wondered why I had worried so over my workload.[3]

A number of mood-disorder patients with seasonal mood changes found out about the NIMH group and sought out Rosenthal and the other scientists working on seasonal mood disorders. One was a woman who experienced regular winter depressions characterized by low mood and the development of an intense craving for sweets and starches. She had made an important observation during the two winters before she came to NIMH: during both these winters, she had taken vacations in the Virgin Islands. On both occasions traveling south toward the equator—to a latitude where the winter days were significantly *longer*—resulted in a dramatic improvement in her mood. Further, the improvement vanished abruptly when she returned to her colder—and darker—home up north. It was becoming obvious to the NIMH team that the crucial factor in seasonal mood changes was *light.*

The word *photoperiod* refers to the length of daylight hours in the twenty-four-hour day. It has been known for many years that photoperiod has a profound effect on many living things. If you've ever put a poinsettia plant or Christmas cactus in a dark closet to coax it into bloom for the holidays, you've used photoperiod manipulation to influence the plant's physiology. The shortened photoperiod causes the plant to produce hormones that cause flower buds to be set.

One member of the NIMH team suggested trying to treat winter depressions by artificially lengthening the photoperiod. Several patients volunteered to sit in front of bright lights for several hours before dawn and several more after sunset. Within three days the first patient began to feel better. "The change was dramatic and unmistakable," Rosenthal later wrote.[4] Phototherapy had been born.

Biological Clocks

In the 1920s the great psychobiologist Curt P. Richter—whom some consider to be the father of chronobiology—started investigating "biological timing devices" in laboratory rats.[5] (He was still pursuing this area of research in the 1980s as a small, stooped but bright-eyed man of ninety-something whom I would see walking through the halls of Johns Hopkins' Phipps Psychiatric Clinic with his battered leather briefcase in hand.)

Dr. Richter recorded the daily activity levels of his rats by putting them in individual cages with revolving drums similar to the wheels you see in pet hamster cages. Each rat's drum was connected to a device that continuously recorded its turnings, providing extremely accurate and totally objective measurements of each rat's activity level on a twenty-four-hour-a-day basis for as long as Richter cared to continue the observations. Each day the windowless laboratory's lights were switched on at 6 A.M. and off at 6 P.M. Richter noticed that his rats, as rats are wont to do, became active and started their exercise wheels spinning shortly after the lights went out, slowed down shortly before their artificial "morning" began at 6 A.M., and slept during most of the day. But his cleverly designed measuring devices were so accurate that they allowed Richter to make another very interesting observation: each rat's activity schedule was almost *precisely* the same night after night. One rat might start his nightly exercises minutes after "lights out" and continue until 4 A.M. while another didn't get going until, say, an hour after "nightfall" and then continued until 5:30. But whatever an individual rat's schedule was, he stuck to it night after night, often not varying by more than a few minutes. Now, since Dr. Richter had not equipped his rats' cages with tiny wall clocks, he concluded that each rat must have his own *internal* clock—one that kept very good time.

But what if the light/dark cues were eliminated? Would the internal clocks still run properly? At first Richter tried keeping the rats in total darkness by darkening the lab all the time. This proved increasingly impractical: a technician or janitor switching the lights on at the wrong time might ruin weeks or even months of work. To eliminate this or any other possibility of light contamination, the rats were surgically blinded. What happened next was remarkable: "The rats continued for some days or weeks to start running at exactly the same time each day, just as if they could still see, [but] sooner or later [they] started running either earlier or later day after day *by strikingly constant intervals.*"[6]

Each rat's internal clock continued to keep excellent time; the trouble was, it wasn't exactly a twenty-four-hour clock. A particular rat's internal clock might have, say, a cycle of twenty-three hours and fifty-five minutes. This particular rat would start waking up five minutes earlier every night, and the rat's sleep/wake cycle would shift in relation to the twenty-four-hour cycle by five minutes a day. As Richter discovered, each blinded rat's internal clock kept to a twenty-four-hour cycle for a while, but then the rat's *internal* clock started keeping to its own particular variation on the twenty-four-hour theme, and the rat's activity schedule started shifting.

Since the internal clock of the rat didn't quite keep a twenty-four-hour cycle, the internal clocks of the normal rats (the rats that could see normally) must have been "set" every once in a while in order for them to be accurately synchronized within a twenty-four-hour day. Obviously the "setting" mechanism was exposure to light. That burst of bright light at 6 A.M. every day when the laboratory lights went on accurately tuned the normal rat's clock to a twenty-four-hour day.

The blinded rat's internal clock no longer kept to a twenty-four-hour schedule because it had lost what we now call its *zeitgeber,* a German word that means "time giver." The blinded rat's internal clock could no longer be *entrained* (brought onto schedule, or reset) by its external "setting" signal: light.

Now fast-forward to Manchester, England, in the mid-1990s. Fourteen healthy young men and women have volunteered for a biological-clock experiment. The vocabulary of chronobiology had changed a bit, the "internal timing device" now being called an "endogenous circadian pacemaker." (*Endogenous* means "inner" or "internal," and *circadian* is a word that refers to a

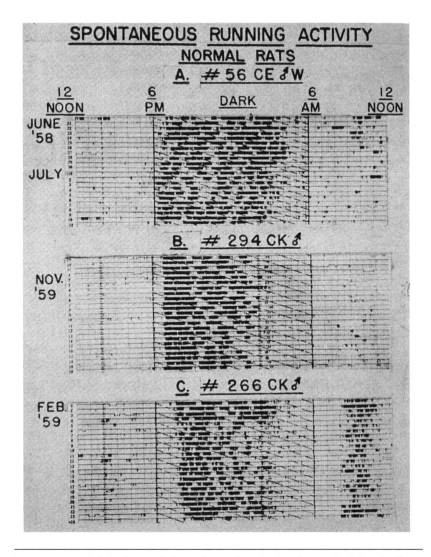

FIGURE 16-1 Original records from three of Dr. Richter's rats. Each line in the records represents one day, the lines becoming thicker when the rat becomes active. Rat A starts running in his cage at exactly 6 P.M. every evening, rat B starts about an hour later, and rat C a bit later still. The records illustrate the remarkable consistency of each animal's internal clock and activity schedule.

Source: Curt Paul Richter, *Biological Clocks in Medicine and Psychiatry* (Springfield, Ill.: Charles C. Thomas, 1965). Courtesy of Charles C. Thomas, Publisher, Ltd., Springfield, Illinois.

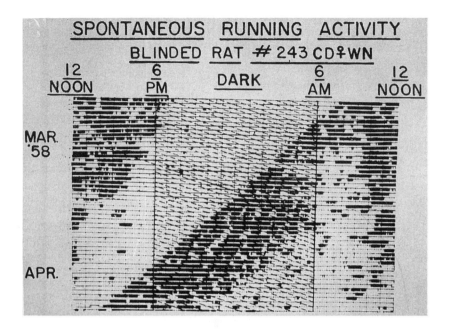

FIGURE 16-2 Activity record for a blinded rat. Each line again represents a twenty-four-hour period. This rat's activity period is shifting by almost exactly thirty minutes every day: the dark line indicating activity starts a little further to the left (earlier) every day.

Source: Richter, *Biological Clocks in Medicine and Psychiatry.* Courtesy of Charles C. Thomas, Publisher, Ltd., Springfield, Illinois.

twenty-four-hour cycle.) Two or three at a time, the volunteers enter experimental living quarters where, for about a month, instead of a twenty-four-hour day they live on a thirty-hour day: twenty hours of wakefulness, ten hours of sleep. Every couple of hours while awake they take a ten-minute battery of psychological tests and rate their mood. What did the mood ratings show?

Here's a hint: like rats, humans also have a close-to-twenty-four-hour internal clock. Although it might be possible to investigate this pacemaker by asking volunteers to live for a month or so like Dr. Richter's rats (in a little room with a cot and an exercise bike hooked up to a recording device), the human endogenous circadian pacemaker can be demonstrated with much simpler equipment. All you need is a thermometer. Our body temperature rises and falls throughout the day, like—well, like clockwork. It is highest at 6 P.M. and lowest at about 6 A.M. Under experimental conditions of constant darkness or dim light, when this clock runs at its own pace, our cycle is about twenty-five hours. But as with the rat's internal timer, our internal clock is entrained by environmental cues, primarily light, to a twenty-four-hour cycle.

Here's another hint: our internal clock can shift only about one or two hours per day. When we reset our watches for daylight-saving time or travel to an adjacent time zone, we hardly notice the change. But when we travel across several time zones, it takes several days for our internal clock to become entrained to the new time. The farther we've traveled, the longer it takes: about one day for each hour of time change.

So what happened to our English volunteers? Since they were forced to live on a thirty-hour cycle, their internal clocks could *never* catch up with their sleep/wake cycle. Their internal clocks started running as quickly as possible but inevitably went in and out of synchronization with their artificially prolonged sleep/wake cycle. The researchers found that the more out of synchronization the volunteers became, the worse their mood became. In fact, it was the *interaction* of the two cycles that seemed to make the most difference in their mood. They felt worst when their internal temperature clock was telling them it wasn't time to get up yet and their sleep/wake cycle was telling them it was time to start winding down from a long day. The researchers proposed that "temporal alignment between the sleep-wake cycle and the endogenous circadian rhythms affects self-assessment of mood in healthy subjects."[7] Put more simply: when our sleep/wake cycle and our internal clock are out of synchronization, it has a very *negative* effect on our mood.

Seasonal Affective Disorder

So let's get back to the patients with winter depressions and summer mood elevations. What can all these findings in chronobiology tell us about the causes of this illness? Do seasonal affective disorder (SAD) patients, with a mood control system abnormally sensitive to light, have some kind of problem with their internal clock? Perhaps a chronic dys-synchrony between various circadian cycles and rhythms?

Several theories for SAD involving circadian rhythms have been put forward, but none fits the experimental findings very well. It had been proposed that people with SAD might have an abnormal delay in circadian rhythms. Early-morning bright light would be expected to correct this problem by advancing the cycle. Evening phototherapy would be expected to have the opposite effect and make things even worse. But research clearly shows that morning and evening phototherapy are equally helpful for SAD. It has also been suggested that SAD patients have lazy circadian rhythms, and even that they are abnormally sensitive to light. But tests of these various hypotheses

TABLE 16-1 Symptoms of Seasonal Affective Disorder

Winter depressions
Mania, hypomania, or normal mood in summer
Carbohydrate craving during depressions
Low energy, sleeping too much during depressions
Reverse diurnal variation of mood (afternoon or evening "slump")

have led to more confusion than clarity, and no one has come up with a theory that ties SAD to a particular circadian rhythm disturbance.

A research group from Columbia University attempted to discover the factors that predicted who would have a good response to photoperiod manipulation. They gave a course of phototherapy to 103 people who reported seasonal mood changes. Some of these individuals met diagnostic criteria for bipolar I, some for bipolar II, and some had unipolar depressions—that is, they had never been manic or hypomanic.

The researchers found that it was not diagnosis (as bipolar I or II or nonbipolar depression) but a particular *pattern* of depressive symptoms that predicted a good response to phototherapy. The people helped by phototherapy tended to sleep more rather than less when they were depressed (hypersomnia) and to complain of low energy and fatigue. They noticed increased appetite during depressions, especially for sweets and starches ("carbohydrate craving"), and an accompanying weight gain. Finally, they had a striking diurnal variation in mood (a consistent pattern of change in mood through the day), but in a pattern that was the opposite of that usually seen in severe depression: instead of waking up early in the morning with the worst mood of the day and then feeling better as the day went on, these people felt better in the early part of the day but had an afternoon or evening "slump," a pattern called *reverse diurnal variation*.[8]

Let's recap some of the symptoms that predicted a good response to phototherapy in this study: a seasonal pattern of symptoms (fall/winter onset with remission in spring), low energy, carbohydrate craving, and hypersomnia. In other words, as winter approaches, these people begin feeling increasingly sluggish mentally and physically, find that they crave carbohydrates, and sleep a lot more than usual. When spring arrives, the symptoms subside. Sound familiar? The similarity to the hibernation behavior of bears is certainly striking.

The serotonin level in an area of the brain called the *hypothalamus* shows a seasonal (twelve-month) rhythm, with the lowest levels of serotonin found in December and January.[9] It is thought that the hypothalamus is the location of our biological clock, and this part of the brain is also thought to be important in the development of SAD.

We also know that serotonin levels in the brain increase after a meal high in carbohydrates. High carbohydrate intake shifts the balance of certain amino acids in the bloodstream and makes some of them, including *tryptophan*, a serotonin precursor, move into brain tissue more easily.

Together these facts suggest that SAD may be triggered by low serotonin levels in the hypothalamus, perhaps related to the short photoperiod of winter days. SAD patients discover that they feel a little better after they have a carbohydrate meal—because such a meal boosts brain levels of serotonin— and they tend to binge on sweets and starches. The fact that the serotonin-boosting SSRI antidepressants are very effective in SAD lends support to this line of reasoning.

But this is in all probability only a crude outline of some of the facts about SAD, and it leaves much unexplained. I've been talking about SAD as if it were a diagnostic category of its own, but it's not. SAD can refer to a bipolar I, bipolar II, or nonbipolar depressive illness that shows a seasonal pattern to symptoms. But a lot of what we know about mood disorders suggests that bipolar I, bipolar II, and nonbipolar depressive illnesses are very *different* illnesses in course and causation. What does it mean that *each* can have a seasonal pattern? The study I described earlier showed that it was not diagnosis but rather symptom pattern that predicted who gets better with light therapy. Does this mean that our whole diagnostic classification system is called into question?

Don't throw out your *DSM* just yet. The "bipolar/nonbipolar" and "bipolar I/bipolar II" diagnostic divisions are still very useful in picking treatments, and so is the "with seasonal pattern/without seasonal pattern" designation. It may just be a few more years before we figure out how all the classifications fit together.

In the meantime, patients with bipolar symptoms who notice a seasonal pattern should talk with their physician about phototherapy, especially if they have the typical SAD depressive symptom pattern: low energy, hypersomnia, carbohydrate craving, weight gain, and reverse diurnal variation of mood (afternoon or evening "slump").

In phototherapy, the person is exposed to bright light in either the morning or the evening, normally using a light-box (similar to the one depicted in figure 16-3). The therapeutic effect is sometimes evident within days, but as with antidepressants, several weeks of therapy are sometimes needed to obtain good remission of symptoms. Side effects are generally minor: headaches and eyestrain, for example.[10] The heat generated by the lights can cause dryness of the eyes or nasal passages. Too much light exposure can sometimes precipitate hypomanic symptoms: irritability, insomnia, feeling "hyper." Fortunately this problem seems to respond quickly to decreased light exposure, and

FIGURE 16-3 Phototherapy

phototherapy doesn't seem to have the risks of mood destabilization that taking antidepressant medication does.

The details of the optimum intensity and duration of light exposure are still being investigated, but several studies suggest that if the light is bright enough, exposure for an hour or even less may be sufficient. The main light-gathering organs of our bodies are, of course, our eyes, and it had been assumed that light falling upon the retinas sends the signal to the brain that resets our internal clock. Some research, however, suggests that the eyes are not the only, or even the most important, means of transmitting light signals to the body's internal clock. A study published in 1998 reported that the circadian rhythms of volunteer subjects could be shifted by delivering a three-hour pulse of light to the back of the knee joints.[11] As with the English study, body temperature was measured to track circadian rhythm. This finding might seem strange indeed at first, but is it really so unexpected to find that exposing the surface of the body, rather than the eyes, to light might affect our internal clock? After all, poinsettia plants don't have eyes, and they can sense a change in photoperiod quite well! It is thought that hemoglobin and other blood pigments may somehow be activated by exposure to light through the skin, in much the same way that chlorophyll, the green pigment in the leaves of plants, is activated by light. This would suggest that the light's signal is carried to the brain by the blood, with an activated blood pigment acting as a kind of "light hormone."[12] Perhaps someday instead of sitting in front of lights during the day, phototherapy patients will strap on fiberoptic cables that deliver light to the backs of their knees while they sleep.[13]

The Sleep Cycle and Bipolar Disorder

We're not finished with circadian rhythms yet. Even if they haven't turned out to explain very much about SAD, circadian rhythms, especially the sleep/wake cycle, are very significant in bipolar disorder. The study with our English volunteers demonstrated how important the sleep/wake cycle is in the regulation of mood in persons who do *not* have mood disorders. So it should come as no surprise that sleep/wake cycle manipulation has dramatic effects on persons with bipolar disorder. Clinical observations confirm this: sleep deprivation can be used therapeutically to treat the symptoms of depression, and it can also cause a switch into the manic state. To understand these observations, we need to take a closer look at normal sleep.

For quite a long time sleep wasn't of very much interest to experimental psychologists and psychiatrists. This may seem odd, especially considering Freud's and others' intense interest in dreams. Possibly because of a lack of investigative tools, interest in dreams never extended to interest in the process of dreaming, and so the physiology of sleep was a neglected area of research for many decades.

This changed in 1953, when a group of researchers used an electroencephalogram (EEG) machine on sleeping volunteers in a clinical laboratory to investigate the longstanding observation that people move their eyes beneath closed lids during some periods of sleep. When the researchers awakened the subjects during what came to be called *rapid eye movement sleep* (REM sleep), 90 percent of them reported that they had been dreaming. Further studies revealed that sleep is a complex process, with several different stages and rhythms of activity that together are now called *sleep architecture*.

As figure 16-4 indicates, after falling asleep a person passes through lighter and then progressively deeper stages of sleep. Brain activity slows, and the heartbeat and blood pressure drop to the lowest levels of the twenty-four-hour day. The process is like a submarine descending into darker, quieter, deeper water. The very deepest stage is called *slow-wave sleep* (SWS) because

FIGURE 16-4 Normal sleep architecture

the EEG shows slow synchronized rhythms in the electrical activity of the brain. SWS is thought to be the physically restorative part of sleep; experimental subjects who are awakened whenever they enter SWS but are allowed to experience the other stages complain of muscle aches and other symptoms of physical discomfort.

About ninety minutes after a person falls asleep, the sleep "submarine" begins to rise again. The EEG indicates a brain activity pattern not very different from that seen in awake individuals. The EEG electrodes that track eye movements measure intense activity, and individuals awakened during this stage report dreaming: the sleeper has entered a period of REM sleep. After fifteen to twenty minutes of REM sleep, eye movement ceases, and the sleeper drifts back down into the deeper stages again and has another period of SWS, which predominates during the first part of the night. As the night progresses, the sleeper spends more time in REM sleep and less in SWS. Toward dawn, sleep becomes lighter and REM periods become longer until finally the person wakes up. It is thought that REM sleep and body temperature are both tightly linked to the body's main circadian clock (often called the *strong oscillator*) because the lowest point of the body's temperature cycle coincides with the most intensive period of REM sleep.

When we look at EEG sleep studies done on depressed persons, the REM cycle seems to have shifted. Depressed individuals go into REM almost immediately after falling asleep, a phenomenon called *decreased REM latency*. Some slow-wave sleep still occurs in the later part of the night, but the overall amount of SWS is reduced. Some researchers have interpreted these findings as indicating that depressed individuals suffer from a *phase advance* of the REM cycle, and that the rhythm of the strong oscillator has gotten out of phase with other bodily rhythms. We saw from the study on the English volunteers that when the strong oscillator (as measured by their temperature cycle) is out of synchronization with the sleep/wake cycle, dips in mood occur. In the few patients with bipolar disorder who have been studied, striking shifts of the REM and temperature cycles were observed as the patients cycled in and out of depression and mania.[14]

These findings bring together a lot of what we know about the symptoms of depression and about circadian rhythms. The decreased amounts of SWS may explain the fatigue and bodily discomfort typical of depression. The shifting of the usual period of REM from the early-morning hours to the early part of the sleep cycle may explain the early-morning awakening typically seen in depression.

These findings may also explain the therapeutic effects of sleep deprivation on symptoms of depression. Patients with the typical diurnal variation of mood seen in depression often report that they have their best mood of the day during the late evening, before they go to sleep, and feel their worst in the morning after they've slept. This and other observations led some researchers in the 1950s to experiment with sleep deprivation as a therapeutic technique for the treatment of depression. With the introduction of antidepressant medications, interest in sleep deprivation faded, but recently it has been growing again. This work shows that if patients are totally deprived of sleep—kept up all night—about 60 percent of them report a sometimes dramatic improvement in their mood. Unfortunately the effect is temporary; in most patients the benefits disappear after even a brief nap, making this interesting technique a not terribly useful one. But experiments with partial sleep deprivation indicate that waking patients up at about 2 A.M. and making sure that they do not sleep during the second half of the night is nearly as effective as total sleep deprivation. Advancing the sleep cycle by six hours, so that patients go to sleep at 6 P.M. and get up at 2 A.M., has also been found to have antidepressant effects.

Although the technique has not caught on in the United States, sleep deprivation and phase advance are popular in Europe as adjuncts to medication in the treatment of bipolar and nonbipolar depression. An Italian study published in 1997 compared the recovery time from depression in ten bipolar patients. All of them were treated with fluoxetine (Prozac), but five were also given several cycles of total sleep deprivation. The patients who had sleep deprivation got better faster on the medication than those who did not.[15]

The other relevant clinical observation about sleep in persons with bipolar disorder is that sleep deprivation can precipitate mania. This is a very well documented finding, and for this reason my discussion of sleep deprivation as a treatment for depression comes with a "don't try this at home" warning: even one night of sleep deprivation can precipitate mania. There have been numerous reports of individuals with bipolar disorder becoming manic after transatlantic flights or after sleep deprivation caused by medical emergencies or family crises. Emotional upsets can, of course, lead to insomnia and poor sleep due to anxiety. It has been proposed that lack of sleep for *any* reason may be what tips the balance for many bipolar patients and brings on an episode of mania.[16]

All of the work on chronobiology and biological clocks indicates that there are important links between bodily rhythms and mood, and we've barely scratched the surface of this fascinating area of study. But so far we have only tantalizing hints about these links rather than clearly understood mechanisms and relationships. Nevertheless, studies of sleep and SAD point the way toward new and safer treatments for certain mood disorders—techniques like phototherapy and sleep phase advance. This work also indicates the importance of lifestyle regularity in controlling the symptoms of bipolar disorder, a topic we'll explore in more detail in chapter 20.

CHAPTER 17

The Genetics of Bipolar Disorder

IT HAS LONG BEEN RECOGNIZED THAT BIPOLAR DISORDER EXISTS IN clusters within families and seems to be inherited in some individuals. In *Manic-Depressive Insanity*, Emil Kraepelin wrote of one family in which "of the ten children of the same parents who were both probably manic-depressive by predisposition, no fewer than seven fell ill the same way; of the five descendants of the second generation, four have already fallen ill."[1]

For many years research on the genetics of bipolar disorder was hampered by foggy diagnostic criteria and a lack of laboratory methods to identify genes. But this is changing. Not only have psychiatrists become more skilled in the diagnosis of bipolar disorder, but the biochemical methods available to locate and identify genes on the human chromosome have become tremendously more sophisticated. These developments will, sooner or later, lead to a better understanding of the genetic mechanisms of bipolar disorder, which will in turn lead to better diagnosis and treatment of the disorder.

Genes, Chromosomes, and DNA

A brief discussion of the principles of genetics, the scientific study of the inheritance of biological attributes, will lead us into our discussion of the heredity of bipolar disorder.

The patterns and rules of inheritance in living things were first described by Gregor Mendel, an Austrian monk who over many years performed elegantly planned and executed experiments with plants, mostly garden peas, in his monastery garden. Prior to Mendel's work in the latter half of the nine-teenth century, it was thought that the traits of one parent were simply blend-ed with those of the other parent in their offspring, who were thought to have traits that were intermediate between the two parents. Mendel discovered that this was not always or even usually true. He found, for example, that crossing a pea plant that produced green peas with a pea plant that produced yellow ones did not produce plants with yellow-green peas (that is, an intermediate form). Instead Mendel discovered that *all* the seeds formed by the cross grew green peas. When he went on to cross these offspring seeds, he found that ex-actly *three-quarters* of the second-generation seeds produced green peas and *one-quarter* produced yellow ones. There were no intermediate forms and no blending of traits. The offspring seeds got either a "green" inheritance or a "yel-low" one; there were no "in-betweens." Mendel concluded that each parent contributed something that determined pea color, and these "somethings" were distributed to the offspring—in this case, seeds—to determine the trait. These "somethings" are now called *genes,* the units of inheritance.

We now understand that genes are sets of instructions for building pro-teins. All plants and animals from seaweed to snapdragons and from earth-worms to elephants are constructed of and operate by means of proteins. Myosin (muscle protein), hemoglobin (the oxygen-carrying protein of red blood cells), and collagen (the structural protein of skin and cartilage) are just a few examples. Even the nonprotein structural materials of the body, like the calcium salts in our bones, depend on proteins. Proteins called enzymes di-rect the manufacture of bone from calcium salts by expediting certain chem-ical reactions. Many hormones are proteins (insulin, for example), and those that are not (like testosterone and cortisol) are manufactured by protein en-zymes. I've already mentioned some members of the protein family that are of enormous interest to those studying bipolar disorder: *G proteins* and the receptor molecules for the neurotransmitters are proteins. All proteins are built according to specifications contained in genes.

For many years it was believed that genes were proteins also—that is, that genetic information was somehow encoded in protein molecules. But by the mid-1940s experiments with bacteria had proven that a far simpler family of biochemical compounds, called *nucleic acids,* contained genetic information. In 1953 James Watson and Francis Crick published a paper in the British sci-entific journal *Nature* describing the structure of the most important of these compounds, deoxyribonucleic acid (DNA), and the modern age of genetics had begun.

DNA molecules are long spiral chains whose links consist of four simpler compounds called nucleotides. The four DNA nucleotides, adenine, cytosine, guanine, and thymine (usually abbreviated as A, C, G, and T), are the elements of an elegantly simple code used to write out instructions for the manufacture of proteins. Just as you can write out a Morse code version of *Hamlet* using only dots and dashes, you can write out instructions for building hemoglobin, myosin, collagen, or any other protein using A's, C's, G's, and T's. That's what DNA does. You can think of the physical structure of a gene as the section on the DNA molecule that codes for one protein.

When the DNA molecule is doing its work in the cell, it is unraveled and stretched out, surrounded by a whole retinue of ultramicroscopic attendants busily reading the coded instructions and making proteins. When it's time for the cell to divide, another set of attendants carefully coil the DNA molecule into a compact cylinder and surround it with protective proteins to form the threadlike structures you may have looked at under the microscope in high school biology: the chromosomes.

Genetic Diseases

Sometimes the links from a certain gene to a certain protein to a certain trait or disease are easy to follow (although in medicine, as we'll see, the pathway to the understanding of these links has usually been from the other direction: from disease to protein to gene). Sickle-cell anemia is one disease in which the links are easy to follow. When the blood of sickle-cell patients is examined under the microscope, instead of the normal saucer-shaped red blood cells, abnormal crescent- or sickle-shaped cells are seen. When biochemical methods allowed scientists to look at the components of the blood cells, it was discovered that sickle-cell patients had an abnormally shaped hemoglobin molecule that tended to form abnormal chains within the cell, stretching the normally disk-shaped cells into the characteristic sickle shape seen in the disease.

Because hemoglobin is easily purified, it was one of the first proteins whose structure was completely described (a feat that earned Cambridge University biochemist Max Ferdinand Perutz the Nobel Prize in 1962). It was discovered that sickle-cell hemoglobin (hemoglobin S) differs from normal hemoglobin by only a few atoms, the equivalent of a single substitution in the gene on the DNA molecule. Because of a number of biochemical factors that made the hemoglobin gene especially accessible and easy to work with, it was possible to pinpoint its location early on in the search for genes that caused human diseases. We now know that at one particular spot on the DNA molecule of persons who have sickle-cell anemia, there is an A instead of a T in the set of instructions. An abnormal hemoglobin molecule results from the reading of these incorrect instructions, and the abnormal hemoglobin molecules in turn cause the abnormally shaped red blood cells, which block blood vessels and result in the symptoms of the disease. The pathway from abnormal gene to abnormal protein to abnormal cells to symptoms has been completely described.

Genes have been identified and located in several other human diseases whose inheritance pattern indicates that they are single-gene illnesses. In some cases this has been possible even though the identity or function of the protein the abnormal gene codes for is unknown. Huntington's disease (or Huntington's chorea), the degenerative brain disease that afflicted folksinger Woody Guthrie, is one example.

Most genetic searches now use *linkage studies* to locate and identify genes. These studies take advantage of the fact that genes that are located close to one another on the chromosome tend to stay together when the chromosomes are packaged into egg or sperm cells. Geneticists take advantage of gene maps that show the location of marker genes in these studies. In a linkage study, DNA tests are performed on blood samples from persons with the condition being investigated as well as on samples from unaffected family members. Sophisticated mathematical analysis of the presence or absence of marker genes in affected and unaffected subjects is performed to find an association between the condition and marker genes. If an association is found, the known location of the markers pinpoints the location of the gene for the condition. This method has been highly successful in locating the genes for several other single-gene diseases, including cystic fibrosis and Duchenne-type muscular dystrophy.

But when several genes might be involved in an illness, the problem of gene identification becomes tremendously more complicated. And if the illness takes several forms or is difficult to diagnose, the task becomes monumental. Unfortunately bipolar disorder is all of these things: caused, in all probability, by several different genes, taking many different forms, and sometimes difficult to diagnose.

Nevertheless, in the late 1980s several reports appeared that purported to link bipolar disorder to specific regions of chromosomes. The most significant report concerned an Amish family that seemed to carry a bipolar-disorder gene located on one end of chromosome 11. In this study, the researchers thought they had overcome at least one of the usual hurdles to finding a bipolar gene. This particular family pedigree seemed to indicate Mendelian—that is, single-gene—inheritance at work. Even if there were several possible genes that could cause bipolar disorder, this particular family seemed to pass the disorder on through only one. Mathematical analysis of previously identified DNA markers pointed to chromosome 11, and the statistical significance of the findings appeared solid. Zeroing in on a bipolar gene seemed to be within reach.

Within only months, however, these results were called into question when another team of scientists took another look at the mathematical analysis. But it was the issue of diagnosis that ultimately scuttled this ambitious study. Several of the individuals who had been classified as unaffected when the data were originally collected developed symptoms of bipolar disorder later on. When the new numbers were "crunched," the results fell apart completely.[2]

Linkage studies have pointed to a number of different locations on different chromosomes as possible sites for bipolar genes, but results are still preliminary, and sometimes, as with the Amish study, repeat testing has cast doubt on the conclusions (although work on chromosome 18 looks encouraging).[3]

A team of researchers approaching the problem from the other direction has also been disappointed. Instead of linkage studies, this group worked backwards from a protein thought to be important in the development of bipolar disorder to try to find an abnormal gene. This group looked for a mutation in the gene for a particular G protein in persons with bipolar disorder, but they did not find one.[4]

What We Know

In the absence of specific identified genes or knowledge about what proteins these genes code for, we can talk about the inheritance of bipolar disorder in only a very general way. Children of persons with bipolar disorder have an increased risk of developing bipolar disorder. Assigning a number to that risk is very difficult because of some of the same problems that have made the search for a bipolar gene so difficult, especially problems of diagnosis. But the risk appears to be several times that of the general population, on the order of 10 percent. However, children of persons with bipolar disorder are also at a higher risk for unipolar (depression-only) illness, and when you add this risk in, the percentages go up into the high twenties. This means that the children of persons with bipolar disorder have about a one in four chance of developing some kind of mood disorder, and about a one in ten chance of developing bipolar disorder.[5]

Persons with bipolar disorder need to be alert to signs and symptoms of mood disorders in their children and to get them into treatment if such symptoms should occur. Although we may be uncertain about the details of the inheritance of bipolar disorder, we are not at all uncertain about the importance of early diagnosis and treatment.

The Search Continues

Several factors make scientists optimistic about eventually discovering genes for bipolar disorder. First, the number of identified genetic markers continues to rise. These markers, like signposts along the length of the chromosome, mark particular locations in the DNA molecule. Imagine that your car breaks down along a barren desert highway that has markers every hundred miles. Imagine yourself on your cellular phone calling the highway patrol and telling them that you remember passing the 100-mile marker, but you're not sure how far back it was. That means you are somewhere between the 100- and 200-mile markers. Let's hope you brought some water with you, because it may be a while before you get picked up! Now imagine that the markers are set up every *ten* miles. If the last marker you remember passing was the 100-mile sign, you're somewhere between 100 and 110. Obviously the highway patrol will find you much more quickly.

The same principle pertains to the search for the bipolar gene: the more genetic signposts there are, the easier it will be to find a particular gene. More precise diagnoses will also help, as will the study of larger family pedigrees as well as technological advances—both the biochemical methods and the more powerful computers and software needed to do the mathematical analysis.

But even when genes are identified and tests developed that can look for these genes in individuals, predictions about who will develop symptoms will probably still be imprecise. This is because several genes are likely involved and also because genetics is unlikely to be the whole bipolar story. There are probably environmental factors operating as well to determine who will and will not be affected; psychological and perhaps physical stresses and traumas are probably very important. So even when a gene or genes are identified and can be tested for, finding that a person has a bipolar gene will probably mean that he or she has a much higher chance of developing symptoms than someone who does not have the gene, but not a 100 percent chance. This will raise questions about who should and should not be tested, and who is entitled to know test results. Siblings? Spouses? Employers? Insurance companies?[6]

But finding responsible genes may lead to new treatment approaches that will benefit everyone with mood disorders. Gene identification and identification of the function of these genes or gene products will undoubtedly shed light on the biochemical basis of bipolar disorder. It may then be possible to design medications or other treatments based on knowledge about the causes of bipolar symptoms on a cellular or biochemical level—as opposed to treatments stumbled upon by accident, which have been the rule so far. Genetics research is one of the most challenging but also the most promising areas of investigation of bipolar disorder and holds the potential of truly revolutionizing the treatment of this disease.

CHAPTER 18

Bipolar Biology

IN THIS CHAPTER I DISCUSS SEVERAL CONNECTIONS BETWEEN BIPO-lar disorder and other aspects of the biology of the brain and nervous system.

"Medical" Mood Disorders

It has been known for many years that symptoms of mood disorders can develop during certain medical illnesses. By taking a close look at these illnesses and trying to see what they have in common, we have learned a great deal about the possible causes of bipolar disorder and other psychiatric illnesses that affect mood.

Psychiatrists used to use the term *organic* to describe mental symptoms that were caused by medical (as opposed to psychiatric) illnesses. Whereas symptoms like hallucinations or mood changes can be caused by psychiatric illnesses like schizophrenia or bipolar disorder, they can also be caused by reactions to pharmaceuticals or by medical problems like epilepsy, hormone imbalances, or brain tumors. When a mental symptom was caused by this latter type of problem—one that could be diagnosed with blood tests or x-rays—psychiatrists designated it an "organic" symptom or syndrome. The implication of this diagnostic system was that "organic" symptoms were not really psychiatric but rather "physical" problems. The other implication was that illnesses like bipolar disorder and schizophrenia—for which, remember, no one could find a physical basis in the brain or nervous system—weren't brain diseases after all but mysterious psychological maladjustments instead.

Now, of course, we realize that illnesses like major depression and bipolar disorder are "real" medical illnesses too and are caused by disturbances in brain physiology. We just aren't yet able to test for and measure the underlying physiological disturbances that we know must be there. Therefore the word *organic* has been dropped from the psychiatric vocabulary. We have new terminology to talk about patients who have psychiatric symptoms that are clearly related to nonpsychiatric illnesses. Instead of referring to "organic" problems, we now say that the patient has, for example, a *mood disorder due to a general medical condition* (the proper *DSM* terminology). Confused? A case study will help explain.

Bea was a sixty-year-old woman who had suffered a stroke about six months before I first saw her in the clinic. She had worked hard all her life as a nurse—in fact had started out as a nursing aide as a teenager, then got an L.P.N. degree in her twenties and an R.N. degree in her thirties. She had simultaneously raised two daughters, one of whom was now an attorney. Bea had been a few years away from a well-deserved retirement when she had the stroke. She lost her speech and the use of her right arm and leg for several weeks. She had been in a rehabilitation center for several months and had made a substantial recovery. But she continued to be very depressed. I had been asked to find out why.

"Mrs. Washington?" I called from the side of the waiting room. A handsome woman with close-cropped gray hair rose slowly from a chair. A smartly dressed younger woman sitting next to her got up too, though much more quickly, and turned to her. "Mama, do you want me to come with you?" Bea looked at me, then at her daughter, then down at the floor, obviously perplexed. "Why don't you both come into the office," I offered. "I'm sure your daughter will be very helpful and will make you feel more comfortable, right?" An apprehensive look came over Bea's face, then she nodded slightly.

I noticed that she walked with a very slight limp on the right and held her right arm stiffly, but she certainly didn't seem to have much weakness remaining from the stroke. Nevertheless, she walked very slowly and seemed to be clutching her daughter's arm as if she might topple over at any moment. Her slowness and obvious fear of falling seemed out of proportion to her physical impairment—and anything about a person's behavior that's "out of proportion" is always of great interest to a psychiatrist.

Post-stroke Mood Disorders

I should pause here for a moment and talk about what a stroke is. The name is well deserved. It is a sometimes catastrophic medical condition that can come upon a person like a bolt of lightning, striking him or her down suddenly, sometimes fatally. The medical term for what is commonly called stroke is *cerebrovascular accident*, or *CVA*. A stroke is caused by a blockage of one of the major blood vessels of the brain (the *cerebral vasculature*). Deprived of the oxygen and nutrients that are carried in the bloodstream, the sensitive brain tissues swell, various toxic reactions set in, and normal brain function abruptly ceases. If the blockage is complete, tissue death can occur. More frequently, blood flow is not completely blocked, or blood gets to the affected area by way of other, unaffected, tributary vessels; in these cases cell damage, rather than cell death, occurs. We don't really understand how and why some people slowly regain the function of the damaged areas and others do not. Bea had evidently suffered a blockage of the left middle cerebral artery, affecting the speech area of the brain and most of the right side of the body. (Each half of the brain controls functions on the *opposite* side of the body.) Bea had made a substantial recovery, better than most people with similar strokes.

"You seem to have made a lot of progress, Mrs. Washington," I continued. "You must have worked very hard at the rehab center."

"Mama works very hard at everything she does. Don't you, Mama?" her daughter said encouragingly.

"It hasn't done me any good," Bea said with a deep sigh. "Not any good at all. I just wish the good Lord would take me," she said bleakly, with a soft voice and dry eyes.

The younger woman's eyes, on the other hand, were now overflowing. "This is not the way my mother talks, Doctor. This is not the way my mother is. This is why we're here. We want her back."

I leaned over toward Bea a bit and touched her hands. "Mrs. Washington, I want you to squeeze my fingers in your hands. This is a strength test, so I want you to squeeze as hard as you can." I felt a feeble grasp from both her hands. "I know you can do better than that," I said. "Squeeze hard." Her grasp tightened a bit. "Squeeze harder, *squeeze!*" For just a moment her grasp tightened so that my finger joints smarted with pain. Her strength was excellent in both hands—once she put some effort into it. "That's great," I said. "I'm not a neurologist, but I didn't notice much weakness at all in your right hand. It seems, though, that it's hard for you to get going."

"Now that I'm crippled, I just can't do for myself the way I used to."

"Mama, you're not crippled," her daughter said decisively. "The physical therapist said you've done the best of any patient he's seen in a long time. And Dr. Lee said—"

"They say that to be kind, but I'll never be the same."

"It sounds like you've given up hope, Mrs. Washington," I said quietly. Bea looked at her daughter, who reached over and held her mother's hand. Then she looked down at the floor. Silence hung in the room for a moment like a fog. I leaned over toward her again. "And I gather it's not like you to give up." Bea was motionless, silent; another tear trickled quietly down her daughter's cheek.

"Well, I have just a few more questions," I said, straightening up and reaching for a notepad. "But I think we can help you with this problem."

The "few more questions" brought out all the other symptoms of major depression: restlessness and insomnia, loss of appetite, feelings of helplessness and hopelessness. But the most striking symptoms were the frequent complaints of "I can't." Before the stroke this lady's favorite words, it seemed, had always been "I can." There was no family history of mood disorders, and Bea had never suffered from depression before. Clearly this depression was related to her stroke.

But, you might ask, who wouldn't be depressed? After all, this proud and independent-minded woman had suffered a catastrophic illness that had forced her into an early retirement and had left her with a limp. Isn't her depression perfectly understandable?

This view of the matter is the one most people took in the late 1970s, when Dr. Robert Robinson began studying depressive symptoms in stroke patients. Why, people wondered, was this bright young clinical scientist spending his time doing research on something so obvious? As is often the case in science, however, taking a close look with an open mind at what seems obvious sometimes leads to unexpected discoveries. This was certainly the case in Robinson's research on the connection between stroke and mood disorders.

The first indication that the obvious explanation for depression in stroke patients—that their disabilities made them depressed—might not be the whole story had come a few years earlier, when a study appeared showing that stroke patients had more problems with depression than other patients with comparable disabilities.[1] These researchers studied twenty stroke patients and ten patients who had suffered other kinds of injuries, like a broken back or neck, that had caused the same level of impairment as in the stroke patients but without injury to the brain itself. A higher percentage of the stroke patients were depressed. When Robinson and his colleagues studied stroke pa-

FIGURE 18-1 This graph illustrates the relationship between the severity of depressive symptoms in stroke patients and the location of the stroke within the brain. The closer the stroke was to the front of the brain (the further toward the left on the scale), the more severe the depression.

Source: R. Robinson and B. Szeta, "Mood Change Following Left Hemisphere Injury," *Annals of Neurology* 9 (1981): 450. Reproduced with the permission of Lippincott-Raven Publishers.

tients, they discovered that a surprising number of them developed a full-blown major depression eight to nine months after their stroke: 67 percent, in Robinson's original study.[2] There were other intriguing findings: patients who had suffered an injury to the *left* side of the brain were more likely to become depressed than patients who had suffered a right-sided stroke. And the most intriguing finding of all: the closer the location of the stroke injury was to the front of the brain, the more severe the depression (see figure 18-1).

These studies helped pinpoint the types and locations of cells and fibers in the brain that we now believe are important in the control of mood. Specifically, they indicated the crucial role of some structure in the forward part of the left side of the brain. This may seem odd if you remember from chapter 5 that the hypothalamus and other structures deep in the lower part of the brain are thought to be the most important centers for mood control. But you may also remember that these centers do their work by way of a bundle of fibers that project throughout the brain. It is thought that this bundle is affected in the stroke patients who suffer depression. The closer the stroke-damaged area is to this bundle, the more likely it is that the patient will be depressed and the more severe the depression will be. These fibers originate in serotonin and norepinephrine neurons, and we know that these neurotransmitters are very important in mood. Just as a single point of damage to a main electrical line can cause a whole section of a city to plunge into darkness, a small stroke in just the right location can affect important bundles of norepinephrine and serotonin fibers extending into large regions of the brain. The result is a change in brain chemistry that causes a major depression. (You might think that medication wouldn't be very helpful for these patients, but fortunately this is not the case. Antidepressant medications are very effective treatments for post-stroke depressions.)

These patients had all the classic symptoms of major depression, and they were caused by the stroke (they therefore had a *mood disorder due to a cerebrovascular accident*). But what about mania? Can a stroke cause a patient to have a manic episode? There have been a number of case reports of people becoming manic after a stroke, but mania occurs much more rarely than depression. For this reason mania hasn't been studied nearly as well as depression in stroke patients. Whereas people who develop depression following a stroke tend to have damage to the left side of the brain, people who develop mania tend to have damage to the right side. They also tend to have damage to one of several linked brain areas collectively called the *limbic system*. Although the functions of the limbic system are very poorly understood, the experience of strong emotions seems to depend on the limbic system being intact. Persons who have large areas of the limbic system damaged by tumors often experience a *loss* of emotional responsiveness, becoming listless and apathetic. It may be that stroke patients who become manic have damage to some small discrete area of the limbic system that usually exerts control over strong emotions in some way. Damage to these "damper" areas thus results in a loss of control over strong emotions: the euphoria and irritability of mania. Patients who become manic after a stroke often have a family history of psychiatric problems and therefore may have a genetic predisposition for mania that the stroke activates in some way.[3]

Mood-disorder symptoms can occur in other brain diseases that involve the limbic system—Parkinson's disease and Huntington's disease, for example. Individuals who have brain injuries from motor vehicle accidents can also have periods of depression. In all these cases, the mood symptoms are thought to be caused by physical damage to brain circuits resulting in chemical malfunctions and changes in neurotransmitter activity levels.

Mood Disorders Due to Hormonal Problems

Another broad category of "medical" mood disorders are those related to various hormone imbalances. By far the most important hormone systems in

TABLE 18-1 Psychiatric Symptoms of Thyroid Disease

Hyperthyroidism	Hypothyroidism
Irritability	Depressed mood
Insomnia	Drowsiness
Restlessness	Lethargy
Hyperactivity	Poor concentration
Paranoia	Slowed thinking
Poor concentration	Apathy and social withdrawal
Delusional thinking	Hallucinations

the regulation of mood are the thyroid hormones and the adrenal hormones.

The thyroid gland is located just below the larynx (the "voice box") at the base of the neck and secretes several hormones into the bloodstream. These hormones are very important in the body's regulation of energy. Thyroid hormones help control the rate of calorie consumption by the body, known as *metabolism*, and the rate at which calories are converted to and stored as fat. If the thyroid gland is secreting too much of its hormones (*hyper*thyroidism), metabolism speeds up; if there's not enough thyroid hormone (*hypothy-roidism*), metabolism slows down. This "speeding up" or "slowing down" affects emotions and behavior as well and can cause symptoms that can be mistaken for those of a mood disorder.

When a person is suffering from *severe* hyper- or hypothyroidism, the clinical picture is pretty unmistakable. But changes in mood and activity level can be the *only* symptoms of mild thyroid problems. Not only can thyroid disease cause mood symptoms directly, it can also make the symptoms of a preexisting mood disorder more difficult to treat. We have already discussed the link between rapid-cycling bipolar disorder and thyroid disease, and major depression can be very resistant to treatment if there is even the slightest thyroid problem. These are more reasons why it is very important to pay attention to this hormonal system and to test for thyroid hormone levels in persons with mood disorders.

The adrenal glands sit atop the kidneys in the lower back and secrete many hormones, including cortisol and adrenaline, which are also important in the regulation of metabolism. Some adrenal hormones are often referred to as "stress hormones" because they tend to be released during episodes of fright or psychological stress and also after physical injury.

Adrenal hormones have potent anti-inflammatory actions; many pharmaceutical products, such as cortisone, are artificial versions of adrenal hormones. These drugs, usually called *steroids,* are a component in some creams used to treat allergic skin reactions, but steroids are also given orally and intravenously to treat inflammatory conditions such as rheumatoid arthritis, asthma, and inflammatory bowel disease. (Steroid creams do not cause psychiatric symptoms. The creams are formulated so that the medication affects only the tissue it comes into direct contact with. Only minute amounts of the active ingredient are absorbed into the bloodstream.)

Excessive cortisol from adrenal tumors can cause symptoms of agitated depression with suicidal thinking. On the other hand, hypomanic symptoms seem to be more common in patients being treated with artificial steroids for medical conditions. Mood-stabilizing medications are helpful in minimizing the psychiatric side effects of steroid treatment. There have been several case reports of lithium, carbamazepine, and valproate helping to prevent irritability and mood instability in patients taking steroid medication for illnesses like multiple sclerosis.[4]

Unlike thyroid disease, the diseases that cause excessive adrenal hormones are fairly uncommon. Too much cortisol causes many physical symptoms, including a change in fat distribution that causes a distinctive facial appearance, muscle wasting, and changes in skin texture as well as blood-pressure and blood-sugar abnormalities.

As with the study of mood changes in stroke patients, we have learned a lot about the normal regulation of mood by studying these hormonal problems that cause mood symptoms. There are complicated control systems for the regulation of thyroid and adrenal hormone production that also involve areas of the brain. Deep in the brain, the hypothalamus helps to regulate metabolism and our physical responses to stress and illness by means of complex feedback loops of chemical signals to the thyroid and adrenal glands. And you've already heard about how important the hypothalamus is thought to be in mood regulation. These intricate mechanisms linking mind and body are undoubtedly important in the regulation of the complex mental and physical experience we call mood. Better understanding of how hormone problems cause mood symptoms will undoubtedly lead to better understanding of how hormones are involved in the normal regulation of mood and in mood disorders such as bipolar disorder.

Picturing Bipolar Disorder in the Brain

For decades clinical scientists have searched for a way to test for bipolar disorder. As we have developed more sophisticated ways of probing the workings of the brain, we have been able to measure subtle differences in brain functioning in mood-disorder patients, and although none of these observations has yet led to the development of reliable tests, we are nevertheless learning a great deal about the disorder with these techniques.

As we saw in chapter 4, early researchers who dissected the brains of persons with bipolar disorder in pathology labs or examined brain tissues under the microscope found no abnormalities of brain structure and questioned whether bipolar disorder was really a brain disease at all. We now know that it is—but that's because we have learned how to look for and measure abnormalities of brain *chemistry*. Looking at the *structure* of the brain, whether with the naked eye, the microscope, or the x-ray machine, has been unrevealing until quite recently. But now two new imaging techniques are beginning to allow us to picture bipolar disorder in the brain.

The first of these is *magnetic resonance imaging,* or *MRI.* This imaging technique is based on the finding that the atoms of objects placed in a powerful magnetic field absorb energy or "resonate" at characteristic frequencies that can be measured with the proper equipment. In medical MRI scans, the patient lies encircled by a large doughnut-shaped instrument that generates a powerful magnetic field. Sensitive instrumentation measures the different resonances of different tissues: bone, muscle, fat, blood, and so forth, and the signals from each are assembled by computer into a picture. MRI is a very sensitive technique, and even small and subtle tissue differences show up with astonishing clarity.

A number of studies have shown that persons with bipolar disorder have an increased number of unusual MRI findings called T_2 *hyperintensities.* These are small areas of high MRI signal intensity thought to indicate change of water content in brain tissue. Persons with blood-vessel diseases of the brain and several other brain diseases are also found to have T_2 hyperintensities on MRI scans, and T_2 hyperintensities also seem to increase with the normal aging process. But although T_2 hyperintensities are not unique findings in bipolar disorder, they are found in higher numbers in people with bipolar disorder than in control subjects matched for age. In one study, hyperintensities were found 1.6 times more often in bipolar I than in bipolar II patients and twice as often in bipolar I patients as in comparison subjects who did not have bipolar disorder.[5]

It's not clear exactly what these signal differences on the MRI images of persons with bipolar disorder represent. Most of the other conditions in which T_2 hyperintensities are found involve loss of neurons and other brain cells and also the pathological process called demyelination, the loss of the fatty insulating material of nerve fibers. Perhaps T_2 hyperintensities are a result rather than the cause of bipolar disorder; perhaps permanent brain changes occur after many years and many episodes of bipolar disorder symptoms, and T_2 hyperintensities are the tiny "scars" of these episodes. Much work remains to be done to explain the significance of these intriguing findings.

The other new imaging technique that is being used to investigate bipolar disorder is *positron emission tomography,* or *PET.* Positrons are subatomic particles emitted by radioactive materials. The PET scan visualizes tissues where positrons are being emitted. In most brain studies, a radioactive substance similar to glucose—the sugar that is the basic energy source of living things—is injected into the bloodstream, and the PET scanner shows which areas of the brain the glucose travels to. There will be higher levels of glucose where there are high levels of brain activity; brain areas with high metabolic activity thus "light up" on the scan. The PET scan gives a glimpse of the brain at work, a *functional* image of the brain that has been a tremendous advance for researchers. PET scans have been used to discover precisely which areas of the brain are involved in particular language functions, and they have been used to investigate the operation of the brain's visual system. The PET scan is also proving to be a powerful tool for the investigation of psychiatric illnesses.

The most consistent PET scan finding in bipolar disorder is a decrease in metabolic rate in the frontal lobes of the brain during periods of depression.[6] The frontal lobes are thought to be important for complex information processing and integration and are also involved in some aspects of emotional control. People who have damage to the frontal lobes from tumors or injuries have difficulty with complex problem solving and are often emotionally dulled and apathetic, two problems that bear a striking resemblance to depressive symptoms. One unanswered question is whether these PET scan findings are unique to the depression of bipolar disorder. Similar results have been found in patients with unipolar depression; the PET scan may be measuring depression rather than marking bipolar disorder. (A related finding was reported in 1997 in an autopsy study that compared levels of inositol in the frontal cortex of persons with bipolar disorder, suicide victims, and control subjects. Inositol is a molecule involved in the second-messenger system of neurons. This study found that there were decreased levels of inositol in the frontal lobes of both the bipolar patients and the suicide victims compared with the control subjects.[7] This study also seems to suggest that there are changes in frontal lobe functioning in severe depression.)

PET scanning in psychiatric illness is still in its infancy. The metabolic patterns seen in the PET scans of bipolar patients are not different enough from those seen in controls and in patients with other neurological and psychiatric problems to form the basis for a reliable test for bipolar disorder—not yet, at least. But as with the MRI findings, the PET findings show conclusively that bipolar disorder is a brain disease with real physical changes in the function of brain areas that can be visualized and measured with the right equipment.

Viruses and Bipolar Disorder

For many years there has been great interest in the possibility that viruses are in some way connected to the development of psychiatric illnesses. Most of the work in this area has focused on the role of viruses in the causes of schizophrenia, but there is growing interest in the possibility that viral infections may have something to do with the causes of bipolar disorder as well.

Links between viruses and psychiatric illness have been sought in several ways: (1) examining birth records to determine if persons with psychiatric illnesses tend to be born during times when viral infections are more common, (2) doing autopsy studies to look for virus particles in the brains of individuals with psychiatric illnesses, and (3) testing living individuals for immunological evidence of viral infections. All three of these methods have revealed the possibility of a link between bipolar disorder and certain viruses.

It has been known for many years that persons with schizophrenia are somewhat more likely to have been born in the winter and spring months when viral infections are more common. A number of studies also suggest that there is an increased incidence of schizophrenia in children born during times of higher-than-usual rates of influenza, measles, and chicken pox. It has been suggested that viral infection of the developing brain during the third to seventh month of gestation may somehow lead to the development of schizophrenia in some people. Several studies have found that individuals with bipolar disorder are more likely to have been born in winter, suggesting that prenatal viral infections may have some role in the later development of bipolar disorder as well.[8]

Testing for evidence of viral infections by looking for viral DNA and RNA in the brains of individuals with bipolar disorder has become possible with the development of sophisticated biochemical techniques that allow tiny amounts of viral genetic material to be isolated and identified. As you probably know from the news coverage of criminal trials, DNA and RNA are unique molecular "fingerprints" that can identify individuals with great certainty. DNA and RNA can be used to "fingerprint" viruses in the same way. DNA and RNA from certain viruses have been found in the brain tissue of persons with bipolar disorder but have not been found, or have been found in lower concentration, in control subjects. These findings provide additional evidence that viral infection may be involved in some way with the development of bipolar disorder, at least in some individuals.[9]

A third method of investigating the possibility that viral infections are involved in the development of bipolar disorder is to test for antibodies to viruses by means of a blood test. Most blood tests for viral infection, such as tests for HIV and hepatitis viruses, don't actually test for the virus itself but rather for chemical defenders called antibodies that the body produces in response to a viral infection. Each type of antibody is shaped precisely and uniquely to fit the invading organism that prompted its manufacture. The presence of antibodies to a particular virus in the bloodstream indicates that the body has encountered that particular virus before. Researchers using this approach have been investigating possible links between bipolar disorder and an animal virus called the Borna disease virus.

Borna disease, an illness that usually affects horses and sheep, is caused by a virus that invades the brain and meninges (the covering tissues of the brain) of the animal and causes progressive deterioration in brain functioning and, eventually, death. The virus is not known to cause human illness, but antibodies to the Borna disease virus have been measured in healthy humans. Although most animals infected with the Borna disease virus develop the rapidly fatal brain infection, some laboratory animals experimentally exposed to the virus have been observed to develop a persistent but low-grade infection that does not cause rapid death. Some of these animals develop behavior changes that bear some resemblance to bipolar disorder: periods of overactivity and of progressive apathy and withdrawn behavior.

There have been a number of studies testing mood-disorder patients and control groups for the presence of antibodies to the Borna disease virus. Several of these studies have found that a higher proportion of the mood-disorder patients have these antibodies compared with the control subjects.[10] This suggests that, in some patients at least, a virus similar to the Borna disease virus may contribute to the development of mood-disorder symptoms. Perhaps there is an interaction between viral infection and genetic vulnerability that can result in a mood disorder. Other illnesses are known to result from this interaction of genetic vulnerability and viral infection. For example, insulin-dependent diabetes, the severe form of diabetes that usually has its onset in childhood, is believed to occur when a combination of genetic factors and a viral infection brings about an abnormal immune reaction, causing the destruction of the insulin-producing cells of the pancreas. Perhaps a similar mechanism operates to cause some cases of mood disorders.

We now know that bipolar disorder is a "real" illness and that changes in the functioning of the nervous system cause the symptoms of the illness. By investigating mood syndromes that are caused by brain disease (like stroke) or hormonal problems, we are learning more about the biology of mood. By allowing us to picture the brain in finer detail and to visualize the brain at work, MRI and PET scanning techniques are teaching us more about how the brain might regulate mood and about the physical changes that occur in the brain because of episodes of bipolar disorder. Finally, work with viruses suggests that brain physiology may be only part of the picture and that understanding the role of viral infection will also be an important part of understanding the whole bipolar story.

CHAPTER 19

Bipolar Disorder and Creativity

ARISTOTLE SAID, "NO GREAT GENIUS HAS EVER EXISTED WITHOUT some touch of madness."[1] Most truisms contain a kernel of truth, and that of the "mad genius" seems to as well. Scholars who have studied the lives of highly creative people have discovered that there are unexpectedly high numbers of individuals with severe psychiatric illness among them. Clinicians involved in this work have concluded that bipolar disorder is by far the most common of these illnesses. It doesn't require extensive research to come up with a long list of writers, artists, and composers whose biographies indicate that they probably had a mood disorder. We'll begin this chapter with a glimpse into the lives of several of them.

George Gordon, Lord Byron (1788–1824), had periods of fiery expansiveness and hollow despair throughout his life. The recorded observations of his friends and his physicians make a diagnosis of bipolar disorder all but certain in the great English poet. Lord Byron's family history is entirely consistent with the diagnosis of bipolar disorder—suicide, "madness," and murder can be traced back for several generations on both sides of his family tree.

Medical biographers of Vincent van Gogh (1853–90) have speculated for decades about the illness that drove him to self-mutilation and repeatedly confined him to the Asylum of Saint Paul at Saint-Rémy. The episodic nature of van Gogh's illness and the acceleration of its course toward the end of his life are highly suggestive of bipolar disorder. Van Gogh described his dreadful depressions in his letters and was diagnosed with mania by several of his physicians. Van Gogh's family history, like Lord Byron's, seems to confirm the di-

FIGURE 19-1 George Gordon, the English poet usually known as Lord Byron, suffered from severe mood symptoms throughout his life (as did several members of his family). "I must think less wildly," he wrote in his epic *Childe Harold's Pilgrimage.* "I have thought too long and darkly, till my brain became . . . a whirling gulf of phantasy and flame."
Source: Culver Pictures, Inc.

agnosis of bipolar disorder: Vincent's brother Théo described his own struggles with depression in letters to Vincent, and a third brother, Cor, committed suicide. Doubters need only imagine the brilliant, swirling, sometimes frenzied colors and shapes of van Gogh's paintings as visual representations of his moods to clear up uncertainties as to what psychiatric illness best explains this artist's episodes of psychosis.

The Romantic composer Robert Schumann (1810–56) wrote of suicide at age eighteen, but only a year later reported, "I am so full of music, and so overflowing with melody that I find it simply impossible to write down anything." Schumann suffered his first major episode of psychiatric illness in 1844 at the age of thirty-four, but he had written a description of his depressions several years earlier in a letter to his future wife, Clara: "No one knows the suffering, the sickness, the despair, except those so crushed. In my terrible agitation I went to a doctor and told him everything—how my senses failed me so that I did not know which way to turn in my fright, how I could not be certain of not taking my own life when in this helpless condition." Schumann recovered from this episode to write some of his greatest musical works, including three of his four symphonies, but ten years later he suffered another collapse. In February 1854 Clara recorded that "in the night, not long after we had gone to bed, Robert got up and wrote down a melody which, he said, the angels had sung to him. Then he lay down again and talked deliriously the whole night. When morning came, the angels transformed themselves into devils and sang horrible music, telling him he was a sinner and that they were going to cast him into Hell."[2]

A few weeks later, probably in the grip of an episode of psychotic depression, Schumann ran out of their home and threw himself off a bridge into the icy waters of the Rhine. He was rescued by fishermen and placed in the asylum in Endenich, where he died a year later, possibly of self-starvation. As with van Gogh, biographers have quarreled at times about Schumann's diagnosis, but a glance at the opus numbers of his works grouped by year of composition (see figure 19-2) leaves little doubt that he suffered from bipolar disorder. What other illness could better explain these intense fluctuations of productivity, periods of intense creative energy that gave way to psychosis and despair?

The fact that a number of great artists have suffered from bipolar disorder does not in and of itself indicate a special link between bipolar disorder and creativity. There have certainly been many great artists, writers, and composers who as far as we can tell did *not* suffer from major psychiatric illnesses. Johannes Brahms, Schumann's musical protégé, who arguably went on to surpass his mentor's accomplishments as a composer, was as staid and steady a man as ever lived. Brahms took his dinner at the same restaurant in Vienna nearly every day for the last several *decades* of his life, often sitting at the same table and ordering the same items from the menu.

Nevertheless, several researchers who have performed psychobiographical surveys of groups of creative individuals have found that a striking and inordinate number of accomplished artists, writers, and musicians have suffered from a bipolar disorder. Most studies have come up with prevalence rates of between 30 and 50 percent—nearly ten times the rate of mood disorders in

```
                                                              146
                                                              145
                                                              141
                                                              138
                                  142                         138
                                  127                         137
                                  077                         108
                                  057                         106
                                  053                         102
                                  051                         101
                                  049                         098
                                  048                         095
                                  045                         094 136
                                  043                         093 128
                                  042                         092 121
                                  040                         091 119
                                  039                         086 117
                                  036                         085 144 116
                                  035                         082 130 113
                                  034                         079 129 112 143
                                  033                         078 125 111 134
                                  031                         076 097 110 133
                                  030 120                     075 096 109 148 132
                              032 029 064          072    084 115 074 090 107 147 131
         124                  021 027 054          060    080 081 073 089 105 140 126
         004         022 017  018 026 052 047      058    065 071 070 088 104 139 123
         003 010 011 014 012 016 025 038 044 050   065 061 063 068 069 087 103 135 118
 007 001 002 005 099 009 013 006 015 024 027 041 046   055 059 062 066 067 083 100 122 114
1829 '30 '31 '32 '33 '34 '35 '36 '38 '40 '41 '42 '43 '44 '45 '46 '47 '48 '49 '50 '51 '52 '53 '54
          |                    |                |               |                         |
       Suicide             Hypomanic            |            Hypomanic               Suicide
       attempt             throughout           |            throughout              attempt
                             1840        Severely depressed     1849
                                         throughout 1844
```

FIGURE 19-2 The severe fluctuations of the German Romantic composer Robert Schumann's musical productivity become strikingly apparent when his musical works (identified here by opus number) are arranged according to the year of their composition. Schumann died in an asylum a little more than a year after his suicide attempt in 1854.

Source: Adapted from Eliot Slater and Alfred Meyer, "Contributions to a Pathology of the Musician Robert Schumann," *Confinia Psychiatrica* 2 (1959): 65–94. Reproduced with the permission of S. Karger, AG, Basel.

the general population. Perhaps the most careful of these studies has been done by Kay Redfield Jamison, who examined autobiographical and biographical materials and, when available, the medical records of all major British and Irish poets born between 1705 and 1805. Jamison concluded that over half of these writers suffered from a mood disorder, more than one-third from bipolar disorder. These numbers are so high that one can't help but wonder if there might be some bias in the research method: do the more tumultuous biographies of psychiatrically ill artists result in more biographical material being available, thus skewing the results? Studies of living writers, musicians, and artists picked by virtue of their having won literary and artistic prizes have been done to get around this possible problem—and have come up with virtually the same numbers. The prevalence of bipolar disorder is simply much higher in groups of accomplished artists than in the general population.[3]

How can this striking finding be explained? Emil Kraepelin thought that manic-depressive illness could free a person from the inhibitions that might otherwise stifle creativity: "The volitional excitement which accompanies the disease may . . . set free powers which are otherwise constrained by all kinds of inhibition[s]."[4] Fear of failure, sensitivity to criticism, worry that one has nothing important to contribute—these kinds of inhibitions will, of course, vanish during periods of hypomania and mania.

One can argue that the extraordinary mental states experienced by persons with bipolar disorder provide them with rich raw materials for the production of works of great creativity. As I tried to make clear in chapter 1 of this book, the clinical states of mania and major depression often bear little re-

TABLE 19-1 Artists, Writers, and Composers with Bipolar Disorders

Artists
  Paul Gauguin
  Vincent van Gogh*
  Mark Rothko*

Writers
  William Blake
  Lord Byron
  Ernest Hemingway*
  Robert Lowell*
  Sylvia Plath*
  Anne Sexton*
  Virginia Woolf*

Composers
  Hector Berlioz
  George Frederick Handel
  Robert Schumann*
  Hugo Wolf*

*Attempted or committed suicide.

semblance to normal mood states. They are not simply exaggerations of normal happiness and sadness but rather are normal moods transcended and transformed. Is it any wonder, then, that those who endure them have put such great effort into chronicling and communicating these remarkable experiences? Because of the relapsing and remitting course of the illness, a person who has recovered from mania or major depression can record what it was like. Individuals in the midst of an episode will usually be too disorganized or too lethargic to be very productive, but later, when their mood state returns to normal, they can express these almost inexpressible feelings and experiences in art, music, and poetry.

It has been suggested that the changes in thinking patterns that occur during the hypomanic and manic states are especially conducive to creative endeavor. When the thinking processes of highly creative individuals (with or without mood disorders) have been studied, it has been found that their thinking tends to be very fluid and divergent. Ideas spring from and give rise to other ideas only loosely connected by logic and convention. Unrelated ideas are merged and mingled in novel ways. Loss of logical progression in thinking and increased flow of loosely connected ideas are, of course, a fundamental aspect of the hypomanic state.

It has also been suggested that it is not any one mood state, normal or abnormal, that gives rise to the creative powers of these artists, but rather the flux and tensions between the different mood states. Constant changes in mood and temperament give the individual with cyclothymic mood changes a kaleidoscopic view of the world, always changing, always new. Perhaps bipolar disorder stimulates creativity in part because its sufferers experience the world through the emotional prisms of its many and shifting moods, some of them extreme, even violent. As the English poet John Keats observed, "What shocks the virtuous philosopher delights the chameleon poet."[5]

Individuals with bipolar disorder may be drawn to creative endeavors out of a need to understand and heal themselves through art and the act of creation. The French author and filmmaker Jean Cocteau said, "Art is science made clear."[6] When medicine and psychiatry fail to explain the inner experiences of the disease, when lithium and antidepressants and therapy all flounder and the terrible moods return again and again, people can find ways of understanding and transforming their suffering through poetry, music, and painting.

All these reasons help us to understand why this terrible and often destructive illness can also generate such intense creativity and artistic accomplishment. If creative work requires unique experiences, fluid imagination, confidence in one's abilities, and energetic excitement about the act of creation, bipolar disorder would seem to fit the bill.

But reading the biographies of these bipolar artists reveals the terrible price they often paid. Bipolar disorder was a mighty but malignant muse for Vincent van Gogh and Ernest Hemingway and Sylvia Plath, all of whom committed suicide. How many more symphonies would Robert Schumann have composed if, like his quiet, steady friend Brahms, he had lived into his sixties?

Perhaps the most intriguing question about the connection between bipolar disorder and creativity is whether or not the illness was somehow *essential* to the creative powers of these individuals. Van Gogh might have lived to paint many more paintings if he had not suffered from bipolar disorder, but would they have been great paintings? Would he have been a painter at all? Or would he have acquiesced to his father's wishes and contentedly applied himself to becoming a member of the clergy? This is, of course, an unanswerable question when historical figures are involved, but a related question poses a very real dilemma for many individuals with bipolar disorder and their physicians. Does the treatment of bipolar disorder with mood-stabilizing medication suppress creativity and dull the artistic spirit?

Several studies attempting to answer this question were done just after the introduction of lithium as a treatment for bipolar disorder in the 1970s (one of them by Morgans Schou, who, as you may remember from chapter 4, was a pioneer in lithium's use as a mood stabilizer). Artists and writers were asked whether they thought treatment with lithium had increased, decreased, or had no effect on their productivity. The results are fairly unequivocal and perhaps a little surprising. Over half (57 percent) reported that treatment of their mood disorder with lithium had *increased* their artistic productivity, and another 20 percent thought it had not affected their artistic output. Only one-quarter of these artists and writers felt that lithium had adversely affected their work.[7] Since one of the side effects of lithium in some persons is a dulling of thinking, it is also possible that these individuals were reporting the impact of a medication side effect rather than the impact of mood stabilization. Would artists treated with valproate or carbamazepine have reported the same results?

Over the years a very few of my patients have resisted taking mood stabilizers because they felt that their creative powers would be or actually were adversely affected by these medications. I have usually thought that these individuals were reluctant to take medications for other reasons: reluctance to accept a diagnosis of bipolar disorder, ambivalence about taking a medication that they felt would "control" them, and other understandable concerns that can usually be resolved with therapy and counseling (see chapter 20 for more discussion of these issues). People seize upon all kinds of reasons not to take medication; my impression is that this particular plausible-sounding reason is usually a substitute for facing and working through understandably conflicted feelings about taking medication.

The mysterious link between bipolar disorder and creativity, though unexplained by either psychiatrists or philosophers, is real. It poses challenges for patients and dilemmas for clinicians, and offers opportunities for researchers. Better understanding of this connection will not only expand our understandings of mood disorders but will perhaps lead us to new insights into the magic of artistry and the creative process.

PART IV

GETTING BETTER
AND STAYING WELL

There are millions of people living with bipolar disorder today. Many are living healthy, happy, and productive lives, but many others are not. This section of the book is intended to help you to maximize your chances of getting into and staying in the first category and staying out of the second.

If you're looking for a simple list of do's and don't's, I'm afraid you will be disappointed. Instead, in chapter 20, "Living with Bipolar Disorder," I've tried to lay out general principles that underlie the sorts of advice and recommendations that are usually given to patients in the doctor's office or clinic. I hope that after reading this chapter, you'll have a better understanding of why some of the do's and don't's that you hear from your doctor and therapist are so important.

In chapter 21 I have collected some principles for dealing with emergencies and have highlighted the types of emergency situations that in my experience patients and their families often fail to prepare for. It's so tempting to put off thinking about and planning for things we hope won't happen. In this chapter I talk about how important it is not to give in to this temptation, and how easy it is to be prepared for emergencies.

Bipolar disorder doesn't just affect the individual with the diagnosis of the illness. Inevitably, family and friends are affected in countless ways, both directly and indirectly. Chapter 22, "The Role of the Family," addresses this aspect of the illness. In this chapter I go over what family members can do—and just as important, what family members cannot and should not try to do—to help their loved one who has bipolar disorder.

We end with a short chapter that looks into the future and explores some of the exciting possibilities we hope will help us to better understand bipolar disorder, to better diagnose and treat it, and, yes, perhaps one day to *cure* this illness.

CHAPTER 20

Living with Bipolar Disorder

THERE IS NO ONE MEDICATION OR TREATMENT APPROACH FOR BIPOLAR disorder that works for everyone. The symptoms of the illness in a specific person are often as unique as the individual, and treatment must be carefully individualized to each patient and his or her particular symptom pattern. This said, I think there are some approaches and pieces of advice that are always going to be helpful. In fact, the principles I am going to lay out in this chapter are in my experience indispensable to staying well and having the best possible control of symptoms.

Confront and Accept the Illness

There is no cure for bipolar disorder, only treatment and management. It is a relentless illness whose symptoms inevitably and repeatedly return to torment its sufferers. The only way to keep it at bay is for the patient to be relentless as well—relentless about getting needed treatment and sticking to it. No other piece of advice I can give is as important as this one.

Human beings have an almost unlimited capacity to explain away the obvious. People who don't want to confront serious physical illnesses can ignore and explain away even the most alarming symptoms: the middle-aged man with a history of high blood pressure who doesn't pay attention to his repeated episodes of chest pain ("Oh, it's just heartburn; must have been something I ate"), the woman who feels a lump in her breast and tells herself, "It's probably just a cyst, I'm sure it will go away." Confronting a possibly life-threatening illness is perhaps the most frightening experience we can face. Small wonder we sometimes put ourselves through some impressive mental gymnastics to avoid the confrontation.

When there are no *physical* signs of illness, no pains or lumps or dizzy spells, it's perhaps all the easier to convince oneself that the symptoms of illness are something else. I don't know how many times I've had a patient ask if I thought he or she really needed to continue on a mood stabilizer after a manic episode had resolved: "After all, I was under a lot of stress, and I hadn't slept for weeks. Maybe I just need to take it easy." As we'll see, stress can indeed play a role in precipitating an episode of a mood disorder, *but it's not the cause.* Stress doesn't make people manic or send them into a major depression unless they have bipolar disorder. Neither does drinking too much or sleep deprivation or the loss of a job or the end of a love affair or the hundred other things that you can convince yourself explain your symptoms better than a diagnosis of bipolar disorder.

People with bipolar disorder can go through years of denial and anger about their illness. I have seen patients repeatedly stop taking medication and drop out of treatment and explain their repeated hospitalizations, shattered relationships, and ruined finances in all sorts of ways: "My wife has it in for me, she put me in the hospital again." "If my boss wouldn't put so much pressure on me, this wouldn't happen." "I think you need to check my thyroid again, I know that's the real problem." Or in its simplest form: "I don't need this medicine, because I'm not crazy."

If you have been diagnosed with bipolar disorder and you have read to this point in the book, you have almost certainly gotten past a great deal of this understandable denial and anger. This is a tremendous accomplishment and signals a turning point in your recovery. (If you're reading this book to better understand another person with bipolar disorder who hasn't yet made it past denial, chapter 22 is especially for you.) But there's a gap between complete denial and complete ability to confront and accept this illness. Unfortunately people sometimes try to hold on to the notion that nothing is seriously wrong by refusing to take the problem seriously. This is especially easy and especially problematic in bipolar disorder.

In bipolar disorder the patient ultimately determines how well *any* treatment is going to work—because it is the *patient* who puts treatment recommendations into action. It is the patient who will determine whether he or she takes *every* dose of medication, or just 90 percent of the doses, or 50 percent, or even less. The patient will determine whether his or her lithium or valproate blood level is drawn exactly twelve hours after the last dose, or whether he or she gets to the lab ten hours or fifteen hours after the last dose, throwing the results and the doctors' calculations off by 10 percent or 20 percent. The patient will determine how many appointments are kept with the doctor and therapist and how many are missed, and how many are shorter than sched-uled because of tardiness. It's so easy to let your guard down, let treatment lapse in little ways, and convince yourself that missing a dose of medication here or there, having that second beer, ignoring a string of sleepless nights, isn't really important. To do so is to turn away from rather than to confront this disease, and often the turning away springs from ambivalence about the need for treatment: *less than complete acceptance of the diagnosis.* Not to ac-cept, not to confront, this illness puts treatment success in jeopardy, because in bipolar disorder as perhaps in no other serious illness, it is the patient who administers the treatment most of the time.

Imagine that a surgeon is evaluating a patient with recurrent abdominal pain. He or she has done a physical examination and has ordered some lab tests and x-rays. All the evidence points to gall bladder problems, and the sur-geon decides that the best treatment among several possibilities is gall blad-der removal. Now imagine that the surgeon is in the middle of the operation and suddenly says to the OR nurse, "You know, this operating room's getting awfully hot, and besides, I'm hungry. I think we'll cancel the operation. I'll give our patient here the antibiotics for another week or so. Maybe we didn't stick with the medication approach long enough after all. Isn't there some new medication that's supposed to dissolve gallstones? Maybe I'll ask Dr. What's-his-name about that. But I just don't think I want to go on with this operation right now."

Sound far-fetched? (I certainly hope so!) Well, here's another scenario: A man with bipolar disorder has driven off with the family for their three-week vacation. The family has already traveled fifty miles when the wife says, "Hon-ey, I packed Timmy's asthma medicine, but I didn't see your medication bot-tle in the cabinet; did you remember to bring your lithium?" The man realizes that he didn't. "Ah . . . sure I did," he tells his wife, and then says to himself, "Three weeks won't make any difference. Besides, I haven't felt depressed or anything in a long time. This is a vacation, after all. And if I get just a little high, it would be OK; I'm sure I could handle it."

Now, what do these scenarios have in common? In both cases, a treatment plan had been decided upon, presumably after much consideration and discus-sion as to the best course of action. In both cases, something comes up that makes continuing with the treatment a bit inconvenient. In both cases, rather than make a rational decision about the best course of action, the person in charge of the treatment uses flimsy logic—accompanied perhaps by a large measure of preexisting ambivalence about the treatment being the correct one in the first place—to justify doing what's easiest. Add in some misinforma-tion—there *is* no medication that dissolves gallstones; three weeks without lithium *can* make a difference, and nobody can just "handle" evolving mania—and you have a recipe for disaster. No one would go back to a physician who treated him or her this way, and no one should treat himself or herself this way, either.

I am suggesting that making a commitment to treatment means (1) being active, not passive, in formulating a treatment plan with your providers, (2) taking charge of treatment implementation 100 percent of the time, and (3) making the decision that you will do everything possible to take control of this illness rather than be controlled by it.

But can a person be "on guard" all the time? In fact, who would *want* to be? What kind of life is it to be constantly worrying about one's mental health? A terrible one, of course. But worrying all the time is certainly not what I'm suggesting. Rather, accepting and confronting this illness means deciding to do whatever you need to do to be as healthy as you can possibly be. This means sticking with treatment and being frank and open with the treatment professionals. It also means more self-discipline and restraint than perhaps you're used to; it means making some lifestyle changes that I'll call *mood hygiene.*

Practice Mood Hygiene

Hygiene is a word that we perhaps don't use in medicine as much as we should, and we certainly don't use it as much as we used to. Hygeia was the Greek goddess of health, the daughter—or in some versions of the story, the wife—of Asclepias, the god of medicine.

Hygiene, or hygienics, is the science of *the establishment and maintenance of health*—as opposed to the treatment of disease—and concerns itself with conditions and practices that are conducive to health. The hygienic conditions and practices we think of today usually have to do with cleanliness, but the word really has a much broader meaning. Institutions like the Johns Hopkins University School of Hygiene and Public Health (founded in 1916) and the London University School of Hygiene and Tropical Diseases (1924) were founded to study methods for *preventing* disease and for promoting and improving the health of whole communities. Predating them both was the Mental Hygiene Association, founded in 1909 by former asylum inmate Clifford Beers (who probably had bipolar disorder). Now called the Mental Health Association, its purpose is to promote emotional health and well-being and to lobby for better and more readily available treatment for psychiatric illnesses.

So, what do I mean by *mood hygiene?* Simply put, practices and habits that promote good control of mood symptoms in persons with bipolar disorder. Several areas of research on bipolar disorder show just how important preventive measures can be for improving symptom control in bipolar disorder. Things like stress management and lifestyle regularity make a big difference.

There is a lot of research that lends support to the *kindling* hypothesis in

Figure 20-1 Hygeia, the Greek goddess of health
Courtesy of the National Library of Medicine

bipolar disorder. Emil Kraepelin noticed that early in the course of his manic-depressive patients' illnesses, their mood episodes often came on after a stressful event in their lives: "In especial, the attacks begin not infrequently after the illness or death of near relatives . . . Among other circumstances there are occasionally mentioned quarrels with neighbors or relatives, disputes with lovers . . . excitement about infidelity, financial difficulties . . . We must regard all alleged injuries as possible sparks for the discharge of individual attacks."

Kraepelin was quick to point out that these events were triggers, not causes, and that "the real course of the malady must be sought in permanent internal changes which . . . are innate." Kraepelin noticed, however, that later in the course of the illness, attacks occurred "wholly without external influences," and he proposed that for patients at that stage of the illness "external influence[s] . . . must not be regarded as a necessary presupposition for the appearance of an attack."[1]

These observations have been borne out in later studies: initial and early mood episodes in patients with bipolar disorder are often related to psychological stressors, but after several episodes the illness can take on a life of its own, and episodes are more likely to arise spontaneously. This is now called the *kindling* phenomenon in bipolar disorder: a match held to a pile of wood will often start a small flame that quickly dies out, but if the process is repeated often enough, a fire is kindled, and no more matches are needed. An interesting parallel phenomenon is seen in animal experiments. An epileptic seizure can be triggered in an animal by applying a small electrical current to its brain. If this is repeated often enough, the animal will start having seizures even *without* the electrical stimulation. Seizures have been *kindled.*

Another interesting parallel in animals can be demonstrated by repeatedly giving animals small doses of stimulants such as cocaine. Over time, animals become *more* rather than less sensitive to the stimulant, and repeatedly giving the same small dose causes *increasing* amounts of behavioral stimulation in the animal. When these animals' brain cells are closely examined, it is found that a certain gene that had not been active previously had been turned on by the repeated stimulant exposure. This same gene can be made to turn on by stressing the animals—by depriving them of water, for example. This work with animals, showing that electrical and chemical stimulation as well as stress can bring about long-term changes in behavior—possibly through alterations in gene function—is thought by many experts to be highly relevant to the study of bipolar disorder.[2] One piece of evidence cited in support of this line of thinking is the observation that anticonvulsant medications, which have "antikindling" effects, are highly effective in treating bipolar disorder.

Several direct observations on patients indicate that kindling may occur in individuals with bipolar disorder: (1) Patients sometimes show more environmentally triggered mood episodes at first in the course of their illness and more spontaneously occurring episodes later. (2) They sometimes show an acceleration in their illness as they age, with episodes occurring more and more frequently as time goes on. (3) Mood episodes make patients more sensitive to stress and more likely to relapse than they might otherwise be. In a study of fifty-two patients with bipolar disorder followed for two years, those who relapsed during the time of the study were much more likely to have experienced some stressful event. In this group of patients, those with a greater number of prior episodes were *more* sensitive to these stresses: they were more likely to relapse under stress, and they relapsed more quickly.[3]

These observations mean several things for persons with bipolar disorder: (1) psychological stress can make a person with bipolar disorder more vulnerable to having a mood episode, and (2) as the person has more and more episodes, the symptoms can be triggered by smaller and smaller amounts of stress. However, (3) there may be a "point of no return" where the illness has become sufficiently "kindled" that stress management no longer has much of an impact, and episodes occur spontaneously and more and more frequently.

All of this means that one of the foundations of mood hygiene needs to be *relapse prevention*. And there should be no doubt in your mind at this point that the most effective relapse prevention tool is medication.

Persons with bipolar disorder should make peace with the idea of taking medication every day for the foreseeable future. This is an especially hard thing to do in this disease. The symptoms and the need for medication often start when people are in their twenties or at an even earlier age, when none of their peers have to bother with medication—when the only people they know who take medication are "old people" and "sick people." It's very difficult for a young, physically healthy person who's feeling well to take medication every day. The idea of taking medication to control one's moods and mental processes is also a daunting one. Remember, however, that in bipolar disorder the medication allows the patient to be in control of the moods rather than the other way around.

Each individual needs to work out for himself or herself a method for making sure that every single dose of every medication is taken. Pharmacies sell a variety of clever devices to help make this happen. There are pillboxes with built-in clocks and timers, with alarms that can be set to go off when it's time for the next dose. There are boxes that hold a whole week's worth of medication in little compartments, one for every dose, so that the answer to "Did I take my dose this morning?" is always clear and certain: if the little compartment is empty, the dose was taken. Or, ask your treating physician if your medication can be taken just once a day, or twice rather than three times a day. Ask about controlled-release forms of medications; a number are available, often making it possible to eliminate midday doses.

The body of evidence showing that medication prevents relapse cannot be argued with; it is simply overwhelming. But there is some evidence that persons who stop medication for bipolar disorder may run more than just the risk of a relapse. There have been a number of case reports of persons who stopped taking lithium for bipolar disorder having a relapse of the disorder *and then not responding to lithium when it was restarted*. Once the lithium had been stopped, it did not work very well for these patients when they started back on it, a phenomenon that has been called "lithium-discontinuation-induced refractoriness." In a series of fifty-four patients who stopped lithium, ten of them—nearly 20 percent—had a poor response when they restarted it. For these patients, lithium had lost some of its effectiveness.[4]

Next on the list of mood-hygiene practices is *stress and conflict management*. Most of us have very little control over when and how stress and conflict come into our lives. But we can learn how to manage stress and conflict better—and here I'll put in another plug for counseling and therapy. This is because I am talking about serious, *vigorous* attention to whatever ongoing sources of serious stress there may be: primary relationship and marital conflicts, job and career problems, and chronic financial or legal problems are good examples. The time of diagnosis with bipolar disorder may not be the time to deal with whatever ongoing and chronic problems of these sorts one might have. But several months later, after mood symptoms have been under good control for a time, would be a good point for some very serious stocktaking, and professional help is highly recommended.

By *stocktaking* I do not mean some process that can be described in a few paragraphs or distilled into the kinds of "helpful hints" and "do and don't" lists that you might find in a magazine article. Rather, I mean *serious examination and fundamental change*. This may involve changing jobs or even careers; selling a house you can't really afford, or declaring bankruptcy instead of struggling with an austerity budget; postponing or reconsidering marriage (or divorce); not going back to school. Just as a person who has had a heart attack would do some serious investigation and hard thinking before taking a job as, say, a high-level manager of a big company, the bipolar patient needs to go through the same process before making big decisions. The stress and strain involved in whatever is being considered should be seriously weighed in the decision-making process.

But serious attention to the "big stuff" doesn't mean that the details of everyday life will just take care of themselves. *Structuring your life* is a very important aspect of mood hygiene as well. In chapter 16 we reviewed the data and studies on the relationship between sleep and bipolar disorder. Remember that a properly synchronized sleep/wake cycle is important to the regulation of mood, and that periods of sleep deprivation precipitate hypomanic and manic symptoms. *Establishing and sticking to a personal schedule* is very important. This means establishing regular times for going to bed and getting up in the morning—seven days a week, if possible.

Research on sleep shows that many other lifestyle factors contribute to or detract from good sleep. Consider cutting caffeinated beverages out of your diet completely, or at least make a rule for yourself not to drink coffee, tea (including iced tea), or soft drinks containing caffeine after noon. Heavy meals late in the day should be avoided. Regular exercise has been shown to benefit sleep and has many other benefits as well on things like blood pressure. *Schedule* your daily walk, your Monday-Wednesday-Friday swim or visit to the gym. Don't exercise only when you "have the time" or "feel like it." Make it part of your regular week, not a luxury.

Don't allow yourself to procrastinate. Putting things off until the last moment invariably raises stress levels. Waiting until the eleventh hour to work on the income tax return and then staying up late tanked up on coffee, searching for receipts and W2 forms, is not something people with bipolar disorder should let happen to themselves. It's no fun for anybody, but for the bipolar individual, it's downright dangerous. File your taxes early, renew your driver's license early, get your car inspected early—you get the idea. Eliminate procrastination as a way of dealing with things, and you've gone a long way toward eliminating a lot of stress. This advice holds true for putting off dealing with interpersonal problems, too. Smoldering tensions in a relationship, chronic conflicts with a co-worker, neighbor, or landlord—these are chronic stresses that will inevitably take their toll on *anyone's* mental health and can exact a higher price on the individual with a mood disorder. Don't put off dealing with these problems, and if you don't know how to approach them, get the professional help you need, whether that means consulting a counselor or a therapist or an attorney.

Alcohol? As I've already said, *the less, the better.*

Some people find it helpful to keep a record of their moods, or a *mood chart.* This can be a journal or diary if you're so inclined, but simpler and less time-consuming techniques can work just as well. If you need to keep an appointment calendar anyway, it's a simple matter to make a notation of your mood every day using a numerical scale. Clinicians commonly ask patients to rate their mood on a 1 to 10 scale, with 1 being the most depressed they've ever felt, 10 the best mood they've ever had, and 5 a normal, neutral, everyday mood. If 1 to 10 seems too confining, use a scale of 1 to 100. It's important to rate your mood at the same time every day to control for diurnal mood variations. Simply record your mood ratings every day by jotting down a number in your appointment book, recording it in your computer time-management program, or marking it on a calendar you keep on your bedside table. Nothing could be simpler, and yet this record will provide you and your clinical team with invaluable information that can help show what medications are or are not working, determine whether there is a premenstrual or seasonal component to mood changes, and, of course, pick up evolving depressive or hypomanic episodes early.

All of this is much easier said than done for persons with bipolar disorder. Regularizing your life in this way may seem quite foreign and strange, not to mention boring. If throughout your life you've learned to wait for the good moods to get things done and just put off thinking about things during the inevitable return of the bad ones, this type of planning and regularity won't come easily. But a growing body of research supports the notion that external regulators like regular sleep and activity schedules help with mood stability.

Build Your Support System

Everyone should have a team of supporters and well-wishers to help him or her get through difficult times. Persons with bipolar disorder are no exception. All of the advice I've given you so far will be much easier to put into practice if you've got a team behind you.

Perhaps the most important members of the team are family and friends. A trusted family member or friend can be extremely helpful by acting as an objective observer of mood changes. One problem that persons with bipolar disorder all struggle with at one time or another is difficulty figuring out which mood changes are normal and which are not. I have seen patients go from one extreme to another in this regard, explaining away severe and obviously pathological mood changes as "normal ups and downs" while they are in denial about the illness, then overreacting and worrying that every period of normal low mood after a disappointment, every enthusiasm over a new project or relationship, means that their medication isn't working. The physician and the therapist can help with this, of course, but someone who is concerned and caring and closer to home can be an invaluable ally in this regard. An astute friend or family member who knows how to communicate observations in a caring, nonprovocative way upon noticing sustained changes in mood is one of the best supports you can have. You may need to give the person you choose permission to be blunt with you. The best person for this task might not be someone who lives in the same house with you; that person may be too close to the situation to be objective. Look around you and choose carefully.

This leads to the question, To whom should you disclose your diagnosis? Two good rules in this regard are that disclosure should be made only to those who *need to know* and to those who *can help and want to help*. The "need to know" category includes, of course, the family doctor, all treating physicians, and any health professional who might be in a position to prescribe medication—even dentists, for example. If you have an attorney or accountant who handles your affairs on an ongoing basis, that person probably needs to know, too.

With employers, things get a bit trickier. If you are asked to disclose conditions you are being treated for as part of receiving medical insurance or other benefits, then you need to disclose your diagnosis. Failure to do so can result in benefits being denied at a later date and claims for reimbursement of treatment costs not being paid. Disclosure up front can avoid a lot of problems down the line, whether this means sharing facts about diagnosis with a new employer or with the current employer at the time of diagnosis. Letting an employer know that shift changes, frequent long business trips, and late hours are things you will not be able to take on because of a medical condition seems to me to be fair to employer and employee alike. As in all relationships, basing the employer-employee relationship on openness and honesty is always good policy.

Although employers are legally prohibited from discriminating against individuals with medical problems in hiring and firing decisions, they can make life difficult for employees they want to get rid of. "Choose your battles" would seem to be good advice here. If you sense hostility at your place of work toward persons receiving psychiatric treatment, it might be doing yourself a favor to look for a different employer rather than for an employment-law attorney.

As for peers and co-workers on the job, the "helping" criterion would seem to be the applicable one, and careful consideration is necessary here. But if you find that you're telling co-workers about your diagnosis in order to get sympathy, to get special consideration, or to get out of unpleasant assignments, you're headed for trouble. There's no better way to breed resentment and conflict on the job. You don't want to develop a reputation as one of those people who use some factor beyond their control to get co-workers to cover for them in various ways. That's not building a support system; it's manipulation, and it will make things worse, not better.

I cannot speak too highly of *support groups* for persons with mood disorders. Under the auspices of several different national support organizations, hundreds of groups provide support to thousands of individuals with bipolar disorder. (See "Resources" at the end of this book for information on these organizations.) Support groups organized by and for individuals with mood disorders and their families not only provide peer support but also are great sources of accurate information about the resources available in a particular community for persons with mood disorders.

I sometimes hear a patient say that he or she doesn't want to attend a support group because "I don't want to sit and listen to other peoples' problems." Certainly, sitting through an hour of whining doesn't sound like something that could be helpful, but that's not what a support group is. Rather, a good support group brings together individuals who share a common problem and who want to learn from each other about coping with it better. It's one thing to ask your doctor about the side effects of a medication that you're contemplating starting, but talking to someone who is actually taking it for the same problem you have provides a very different and a very valuable perspective. Within a support group, you may have an opportunity to ask other persons with bipolar disorder how *they* told their boss or their children about their diagnosis, what *they* do to remember a complicated medication schedule, and a thousand other questions.

Don't Be a "Bipolar Victim"

Individuals with any incurable but treatable medical problem must learn how to walk the fine line between not taking their illness seriously enough and taking it *too* seriously. We psychiatrists see the consequences of not taking bipolar disorder seriously enough every day in our offices and clinics—and, more often than not, in hospitals and emergency rooms. Individuals who stop taking medication, who won't get the treatment they need for a substance-abuse problem, who ignore ongoing environmental stresses and interpersonal problems until they are overwhelmed by them—these individuals are truly victims of bipolar disorder who abdicate to the whims and erratic rhythms of their illness rather than do what they can to control their symptoms. But there's another kind of victim as well: the person who worries about his or her symptoms and illness all the time, who avoids challenges and withdraws from work and the community into a world of medications, blood tests, doctor's visits, and support-group meetings. I think most individuals with bipolar disorder spend some time on both sides of this fine line for a while as they sort out the impact of the illness on their view of themselves and figure out how to integrate what they need to do about the illness into their lifestyle. Neither extreme is healthy, and it takes time, good advice, and hard work to find the proper balance.

Perhaps the biggest obstacle to finding this balance is *stigma*. Sociologist Erving Goffman explained the grisly origins of the word in the introduction to his 1963 essay on the subject, *Stigma: Notes on the Management of Spoiled Identity:* "The Greeks, who were apparently strong on visual aids, originated the term *stigma* to refer to bodily signs designed to expose something unusual and bad about the moral status of the signifier. The signs were cut or burnt into the body and advertised that the bearer was . . . a blemished person, ritually polluted, to be avoided, especially in public places." Goffman had originally become interested in the issues of stigma, prejudice, and discrimination against physically handicapped individuals who had some immediately visible sign of their being different in some way: persons who were blind or disfigured or who had had a limb amputated. He soon came to realize, however, that the same issues were relevant, but became much more complicated, when there was no outward sign of the stigmatized condition, as in "the blemishes of individual character . . . mental disorder, imprisonment, addiction."[5]

Fortunately psychiatric conditions like bipolar disorder are not often considered "blemishes of individual character" anymore, but they are stigmatized just the same. Persons with psychiatric conditions are too often regarded as untreatable and thus unpredictable and dangerous, or at the very least unreliable and incompetent. Too many films and television programs still ridicule or demonize individuals with psychiatric illnesses, and words like *crazy* and *insane* are generalized terms of contempt that you can hear in any schoolyard during recess. Individuals with bipolar disorder have usually incorporated these prejudiced and negative views into their own way of thinking from a very young age. This means that when they themselves are diagnosed with bipolar disorder, they have to deal not only with the prejudices and unfair biases others may have toward them, but also with their *own* negative ideas and feelings about persons with a psychiatric illness. People can react to this in opposite ways, either not accepting the diagnosis and remaining in denial about the illness, or giving in to all of their negative thinking and feelings and becoming "a bipolar" rather than "a person who has bipolar illness," telling everyone and anyone about their illness and using it as an excuse to avoid responsibilities and challenges. In either case, the individual has become a victim of the illness.

How can you avoid becoming a victim? You've taken a big step by getting this book. Accurate information about what bipolar disorder is and is not provides an excellent defense against prejudiced thinking and bad decisions based on misinformation. A close second to getting accurate information is getting the support, feedback, and advice—and the opportunity to ask questions and just vent your fears and frustrations—that counseling, therapy, and support groups provide. No one needs to confront this problem and sort through all the conflicting emotions and feelings alone—and no one should.

CHAPTER 21

Planning for Emergencies

THE DECISIONS WE ARE FORCED TO MAKE IN A CRISIS ARE FREQUENTLY NOT the decisions we would have made under other circumstances. When an emergency arises for which we are unprepared, we are usually forced to improvise a response as we go along. In this chapter I want to identify several potential emergencies that may face the individual with bipolar disorder and his or her family and discuss how to prepare for and deal with them. One of the best ways to prepare for an emergency is to have a crisis plan ready to go.

Because we have such effective treatments available for bipolar disorder, we sometimes forget that this is a potentially lethal illness. And when you are dealing with a disease that has the potential to become life-threatening, the last thing you want is an improvised response to an emergency situation.

I could sense the frustration in Lisa's voice as I listened to her speaking into the emergency-room phone.

"I hear you, ma'am, but the magistrate won't approve a petition for involuntary treatment just because your husband isn't taking his medication. I need more information before we can—"

Suddenly she stopped and put the phone down. "I can't believe it; she hung up on me." Lisa looked down at her notepad, then turned to me. "Does the name Stanley Winters mean anything to you? That was his wife. She wanted someone to come out to their house and bring him into the emergency room. She said he's very depressed."

"The name doesn't ring any bells with me," I replied. "Let's try the computer to see if he's ever had any treatment here before. Maybe we've got some records. Then we can try calling her back." As Lisa stepped over to the emergency room's computer terminal, I glanced at my watch. It was almost noon, and I had a lunchtime lecture to give. "Lisa, I have to go give my lecture to the medical students. If we have a chart on Mr. Winters, can you order it from Medical Records? I'll be back a little after one, and we can see what we're dealing with and get back with Mrs. Winters."

It was just minutes past one when my beeper went off, with a message to call the emergency room.

"Frank, this is Lisa. Mr. and Mrs. Winters are here in the ER. Well, that's not exactly true. Mrs. Winters is here, but Mr. Winters won't get out of the car. Do you think you could come down?"

I hadn't done any parking-lot therapy for a while, and as I walked past the "Authorized Personnel Only Please" sign that guarded the door to the emergency room, I wondered who and what would be waiting for me. I walked into the nursing station and asked the secretary where the psychiatric nurse was. I had no sooner asked the question than Lisa walked in. "I went out and persuaded him to come in. They're in room 5. He's not doing too well; I think he'll need to be admitted. I'll call the unit and see if we have any beds."

"Has he been here before? Were you able to get a chart?" I asked.

"The last time he was here was about eight years ago, so the chart is on microfilm. We should have it soon, but the computer says he was admitted and the discharge diagnosis was bipolar disorder, manic episode."

"Well, that's some help. Let me go see them."

As soon as I opened the door to the interview room, I could see that (as usual) Lisa had sized up the situation pretty accurately. Mr. and Mrs. Winters looked to be in their early fifties. He was sitting in a corner, staring at the floor, and he looked as if he hadn't shaved in about a week. Mrs. Winters was sitting next to him but got up as I entered the room. "I practically had to carry him to get him into the car to come here," she said. "I've been desperate. He hasn't eaten anything in four days. We've only been married for a year, and I didn't realize—I mean, I didn't know how bad . . . I called his psychiatrist's office, but they said she wasn't practicing anymore."

It took a while to get Mrs. Winters calmed down, and even longer to get the whole story. Mr. Winters was obviously in the grip of serious depression and was barely able to talk, let alone give any kind of history of his problems.

When the microfilmed records arrived, they told us that Stan had been treated for mood problems since he was in his thirties. Our records of his treatment for a manic episode indicated that he had done well on lithium during the hospitalization. I recognized the name of the psychiatrist in the records as a colleague who had retired about six months before. I knew for a fact that she had sent letters announcing her retirement almost a year before she quit her practice group.

I was getting the more recent history from Stan's wife when I heard a knock on the door. Lisa peeked in. "Dr. Mondimore, can I see you for a moment?"

"Excuse me," I said and stepped outside. Lisa was holding the "preferred-provider" and HMO list that was posted on the ER bulletin board. "His insurance doesn't pay here. If he needs to be admitted, he'll have to go to Harris Memorial."

"Great," I grumbled. "He definitely needs to be in the hospital, but his wife had a terrible time getting him here. I don't think we should let her transport him. Can you have the secretary call the hospital transportation people?"

Lisa frowned. "Our transportation won't take patients to a hospital outside our system. We'll need to call an ambulance."

"That will cost these folks several hundred dollars. We can't use our people for a three-mile ride?" Lisa gave me her very best "I don't make the rules, I just follow them" look and said nothing. I took a deep breath and prepared to go tell the Winterses that it would probably be several more hours before Stan would be in the hospital.

People usually enjoy making plans—vacation plans, wedding plans, retirement plans. Planning for a psychiatric emergency is much less enjoyable but, unfortunately, much more important. Unlike vacation plans, these are plans that no one would be disappointed about not getting to use. But if you do need them, odds are you'll be very glad you made them.

Mr. Winters appeared to be operating under the assumption that his bipolar disorder had gone away for good (mistake #1). So when the letter came from the office of his psychiatrist announcing her retirement, he put off making arrangements to get hooked up with a new one. When the emergency came along, he had no treating physician familiar with his situation (mistake #2). He and his wife had obviously not had a very detailed discussion about bipolar disorder, about what she should do if symptoms flared up leaving Stan unable to make good decisions about treatment (mistake #3). Mrs. Winters was not familiar with the law and the procedures in their community regarding involuntary commitment of persons with psychiatric illness (mistake #4).

And last but not least, the Winterses were unfamiliar with the requirements of their medical insurance plan and went to a hospital where their insurance would not approve hospitalization (mistake #5).

How long would it have taken to prevent all these mistakes? An hour or two? Maybe three? Obviously this would have been time well spent. Let's review some of the things it is important to know about in planning for this type of emergency.

Know Whom to Call for Help

I've always thought that the people who can handle almost anything are those who know when they need help and whom to call for it. Persons with bipolar disorder owe it to themselves to be under the care of a psychiatrist who is familiar with their symptoms and the course of their illness. This means establishing yourself with a new physician when you move to a new community or if any other factor, such as the retirement of your psychiatrist, leaves you "uncovered." Changes in insurance plans sometimes force a change in psychiatrists. Don't put off making an appointment to get established as a patient in a new community or with a new practice. Because it can sometimes take months for records to be transferred from one office to another, ask if you can be given a copy of your records or a letter of introduction that you can bring to your new doctor at the first appointment.

Don't hesitate to ask the psychiatrist how his or her practice is covered after hours. How easy is it to get a routine office appointment? Are appointments set aside that can be set up within a day or two for emergencies? Every psychiatrist or mental-health clinic should have some means of seeing patients within twenty-four hours in cases of true emergencies. One that does not is one to steer clear of.

Be sure your know how to contact the psychiatrist or his or her office at any time of the day or night and what arrangements are in place to handle emergencies. Does the psychiatrist see his or her own emergencies, or does everyone in the practice rotate emergency "on-call" duty? The on-call system, though not ideal, is often the standard in a practice, meaning that you may well see a doctor other than your regular one if you have an acute emergency. Are you prepared for such an arrangement in order to be under the care of a psychiatrist who comes highly recommended?

What hospitals does your psychiatrist or his or her practice have a relationship with? Does he or she admit to the hospital you prefer? To the hospital where your insurance covers in-patient psychiatric treatment?

If the answers to these questions are not satisfactory, consider your options. Ask your family doctor, family members, friends, or members of your support group for recommendations. Call the local chapter of the Mental

Health Association, the National Depressive and Manic-Depressive Association, or another advocacy group for a referral. (These groups are listed in "Resources" at the end of this book.) Sometimes your options are limited by medical insurance coverage—which brings us to another important aspect of being prepared.

Insurance Issues

Be familiar with the details of your medical insurance coverage for psychiatric illness. Unfortunately most plans treat psychiatric illnesses differently from nonpsychiatric illnesses. For example, they frequently have different and stricter limits on hospitalization coverage, the number of out-patient appointments they will pay for, and the percentage or amounts that patients must pay out of pocket for certain services ("co-payments"). Some insurance plans exclude coverage for treatment of psychiatric illness altogether or provide psychiatric coverage for an additional charge.

Do you have a lifetime "cap" on psychiatric services? This might be a limit on days of hospitalization or on number of out-patient appointments per year, or there might be a dollar-amount limit to coverage. Are you limited to or covered at a lower rate at certain hospitals or practice groups? If your insurance company denies coverage for a hospitalization or for several days of hospitalization, what are the procedures by which you can appeal the decision?

Hospital stays of all types are getting shorter, and psychiatric hospitalization is no exception. Hospitalization is reserved almost exclusively for life-threatening emergencies now, and patients are discharged as soon as possible. Patients are no longer hospitalized in a psychiatric unit or a psychiatric hospital for weeks or months. Does your psychiatrist have access to a *partial hospitalization* program (sometimes also referred to as a *day hospital*)? This alternative to traditional hospital treatment provides hospital-like monitoring and treatment during the day, or sometimes for only part of the day, but allows patients to return home in the evening and spend the night there. It is a very useful treatment option for bipolar disorder because it offers a way to provide daily monitoring of mood symptoms and treatment response without the disruption to personal and family life that staying in a hospital causes. Some insurers cover a partial hospitalization—even insist on it—but others do not. Know where your insurance company and your psychiatrist stand on partial hospitalization.

Everyone these days seems to be talking about "managed care." If you are a member of an HMO, you are part of the managed-care picture. (In a *health maintenance organization,* members pay a monthly fee to receive their medical care from the organization.) But even if you are not in an HMO, aspects of managed-care practice probably affect you in one way or another, no matter what kind of insurance you have.

Managed care means that the organization that is financially responsible for your medical care—your medical insurance company or HMO, for example—supervises or manages how much medical care you receive. This is accomplished in a variety of ways, some of which may be visible to you, some not. The main purpose of this management is to minimize your use of more expensive types of medical care, usually meaning hospitalization and treatment by specialists. In an HMO you may have to be referred by a primary physician to any specialists—including psychiatrists—in order to be covered. Lab tests may be covered only if your primary physician approves them (this can make it inconvenient to get the blood tests needed to monitor therapy with lithium and some other psychiatric drugs). If you are admitted to a hospital, your doctor may be called every few days by someone from the HMO or from the insurance company asking why you still need to be in the hospital, a function called *utilization review*. If this reviewer (usually a nurse) thinks you should be discharged, he or she will tell your doctor (and you) that coverage will be denied after a certain date and that you will be financially responsible for any additional inpatient treatment. (A variety of appeals procedures usually kick in at this point if your doctor disagrees.) Once usually limited to inpatient treatment, managed care is now becoming very interested in outpatient treatment as well, and psychiatrists are being asked to fill out forms specifying a treatment plan and requesting a certain number of office visits.

If the insurance plan includes coverage for pharmacy charges, you may not have a choice of brands of medication but will need to take whatever equivalent generic pharmaceutical the pharmacy stocks. Some HMOs have expanded on this theme and limit coverage to some members of a broadly defined class of medications, not permitting their doctors even to prescribe others. (For a while some insurance would not pay for SSRI antidepressants but would insist that tricyclic antidepressants be tried first.)

There was a time when medical treatment was controlled by doctors and patients. That time has passed. Managed-care methods save millions upon millions of health-care dollars. Some people argue that this means that more people have access to better medical care because the system is more efficient and effective. Others argue that "managed care" is an oxymoron. But whichever is the case, managed-care methods are used commonly in all types of insurance coverage now. Your type of medical insurance will almost certainly determine which hospital you can be admitted to, and it may determine which doctor you can see. Your insurance company will probably supervise the length of your hospitalizations and possibly control the number of office visits you can have, even which medications can be prescribed for you. All of this means that you should closely scrutinize all aspects of your insurance coverage for psychiatric illness, your existing policy and any new policies that you may have to choose from because of job changes. Don't put yourself in the position of getting an emergency-room surprise.

Safety Issues and Hospitalization

The most dangerous emergency situation for persons with bipolar disorder, and one that frequently leads to hospitalization, is the development of suicidal thoughts and behaviors. In studies from the 1940s, suicide rates of 30 and even 60 percent were reported in groups of bipolar patients. Thankfully, the availability of modern treatments for bipolar disorder has greatly changed these grim numbers. Nevertheless, the rate of suicide deaths in persons with bipolar disorder is many times that seen in the general population—in some studies, thirty to nearly eighty times higher.[1]

It may seem obvious to say that the most effective way of minimizing the risk of suicide in bipolar disorder is relapse prevention. But if I had said "*relapse* prevention is *suicide* prevention" in the last chapter, you might have thought I was just being dramatic. Do not *ever* lose sight of the fact that bipolar disorder is a potentially fatal disease: relapse prevention *is* suicide prevention.

Individuals with bipolar disorder should not have firearms in the home. There are any number of scientific studies showing that having a firearm in a home increases the chances of a violent death occurring in that home, either by suicide or by homicide.[2] Where an illness whose symptoms can include suicidal depression and heightened irritability with loss of inhibitions is concerned, there is never, *ever,* any justification whatsoever for having a gun of any type in the home. Period.

The emergence of self-destructive thoughts and impulses is frightening both to the patient and to those around him or her. The tremendous stigma and disgrace that have been associated with suicide for centuries still make people reluctant to discuss these thoughts when they occur. These ideas, and notions like "only crazy people kill themselves," complicate what is really a much simpler clinical issue: suicidal thinking is a serious symptom of this illness, which must be evaluated quickly by a professional and managed swiftly and effectively. Patients can be intensely ashamed of suicidal thoughts and feel that the development of self-destructive impulses is a kind of failure. Of course it is not a failing in any way; it is a symptom of an illness. It is important to see the development of suicidal feelings in a bipolar patient as a very dangerous symptom of serious illness, just like the onset of chest pains in a heart patient. When they occur, it's not time to wonder about what they mean, *it's time to call for help.* And just as with the development of chest pains in a heart patient, the development of suicidal feelings in a mood-disorder patient is often a reason for hospitalization.

Psychiatric hospitalization can be experienced as a terrible failure. Again, the clinical perspective tells us otherwise. Although we have gotten much better at treating bipolar disorder, our treatment methods are by no means perfect. Sometimes, despite everyone's very best efforts, relapses occur and serious symptoms like suicidal feelings emerge and require hospitalization. When this happens, it's not time for self-blame or questions like, What did I do wrong? Rather, it's time for healing.

Remember that the word we often used in the past for psychiatric hospitals was *asylum,* defined as "a place offering protection and safety."[3] Individuals whose will has been temporarily seized by this terrible illness and who are on the verge of terrible and desperate action deserve a place of protection and safety. No apologies are *ever* necessary, no reproach ever justified.

One more reminder: bipolar disorder can raise issues of personal safety. These issues need to be anticipated, discussed, planned for, and promptly addressed if and when they arise. Because family members are often a crucial part of dealing with these emergencies, I'll be discussing these issues further in the next chapter.

CHAPTER 22

The Role of the Family

THE CHALLENGES OF LIVING WITH BIPOLAR DISORDER ARE NOT LIM-
ited to those who have the disease. Family and friends face them as well. It's
intensely painful to see a loved one suffer from the desperate bleakness of major depression, and just as painful and frightening to see him or her in the frenzied grip of mania. As in any illness, the role of the family includes support,
understanding, and encouragement of the person who is ill. The first step in
being able to provide this kind of support is understanding some very important facts about the illness.

Recognizing Symptoms

Never forget that the person with bipolar disorder does not have control
of his or her mood state. Those of us who do not suffer from a mood disorder
sometimes expect mood-disorder patients to be able to exert the same control
over their emotions and behavior that we ourselves are able to. When we sense
that we are letting our emotions get the better of us and we want to exert some
control over them, we tell ourselves things like "Snap out of it," "Get a hold of
yourself," "Try and pull yourself out of it." We are taught that self-control is a
sign of maturity and self-discipline. We are indoctrinated to think of people
who don't control their emotions very well as being immature, lazy, self-in-
dulgent, or foolish. But you can only exert self-control if the control mechanisms are working properly, and in people with mood disorders, they are not.

People with mood disorders cannot "snap out of it," much as they would like to (and it's important to remember that they want *desperately* to be able to). Telling a depressed person things like "pull yourself out of it" is cruel and may in fact reinforce the feelings of worthlessness, guilt, and failure already present as symptoms of the illness. Telling a manic person to "slow down and get hold of yourself" is simply wishful thinking; that person is like a tractor trailer careening down a mountain highway with no brakes.

So the first challenge facing family and friends is to change the way they look at behaviors that might be symptoms of the illness—behaviors like not wanting to get out of bed, being irritable and short-tempered, being "hyper" and reckless or overly critical and pessimistic. Our first reaction to these sorts of behaviors and attitudes is to regard them as laziness, meanness, or immaturity and be critical of them. In a person with bipolar disorder, this almost always makes things worse: criticism reinforces the depressed patient's feelings of worthlessness and failure, and it alienates and angers the hypomanic or manic patient.

This is a hard lesson to learn. Don't always take behaviors and statements at face value. Learn to ask yourself, "Could this be a symptom?" before you react. Little children frequently say "I hate you" when they are angry at their parents, but good parents know that this is just the anger of the moment talking; these are not their child's true feelings. Manic patients will say "I hate you" too, but this is the illness talking, an illness that has hijacked the patient's emotions. The depressed patient will say, "It's hopeless, I don't want your help." Again, this is the illness and not your loved one rejecting your concern.

I'm now going to make things really difficult by warning against the other extreme: interpreting *every* strong emotion in a person with a mood disorder as a symptom. This other extreme is just as important to guard against. I have seen many couples in which one partner has a bipolar disorder and the healthy partner wields the diagnosis as a weapon to emotionally subdue the other. (Come to think of it, that doesn't sound very "healthy," does it?)

"Vicky's medication needs an adjustment. I'm sure of it."

Vicky stared down at the floor angrily as Peter went on. "She won't give up on this crazy idea about going back to college." I winced a little at Peter's use of the word *crazy,* a word that can make a person with a psychiatric illness feel like they've just been slapped in the face. I made a mental note to bring it to his attention later, but to do so now might make it look as if I was "taking sides."

"Peter," I said, "I'd like to hear from Vicky about this. She's been doing well for over two years now; I think it may be time to have a serious discussion about her idea."

Vicky looked up. "I was six months away from graduating from Bryn

Mawr when I got sick the first time. I've called State, St. James College, and Everett, and I could get my degree with only a year of study at any of them."

Vicky was in her mid-thirties, an intense, vibrant woman who I suspected was probably brilliant as well. Peter had been transferred to town by his company a month after Vicky had gotten out of the hospital following a nearly lethal suicide attempt. It had taken three hospitalizations for her to be properly diagnosed as having bipolar disorder—after nearly ten years of roller-coaster moods. She had been treated for a depressive disorder, for a personality disorder, even for schizophrenia before she started on valproate and had a big turnaround. She had done so well, in fact, that I had seen her only half a dozen times over the past two years. About half the time her husband came along to her appointments. Every couple of months I noticed a book review she had written in the local newspaper, and on one visit she had mentioned working on a biography of Mary Todd Lincoln. Going back to college seemed well within her capabilities.

Peter sighed, then went on. "It makes me really nervous to see her up late at night looking at college entrance requirements over the Internet. And we've gotten dozens of college catalogs through the mail that she's called or written for. I'm afraid she's getting manic, and I just can't go through that again."

Vicky's eyes flashed, and she drew in her breath, then slowly released it. "Peter's not used to me being this confident and energized about anything. We've only been married for four years, and for nearly two of those I was more or less depressed. This is me, not mania." Her voice became just the slightest bit louder. "But he's treating me like a child, an incompetent." She looked over at her husband. "A lunatic, right? I'm finally getting back to *my* goals and career after ten years, and what did you call it? 'Crazy'?"

Now it was Peter's turn to look angry. "You see, Doctor? Do you see what I mean, how angry she gets? She's not usually like this. Before we came here today, she—"

"Oh, God, stop it." Vicky said quietly, through clenched teeth. Tears were flowing now.

"OK, you two, let's cool down for a moment," I said. I could sense that this was a continuation of a power struggle between Peter and Vicky that had probably been going on for weeks, maybe even months. But I also had the sense that Vicky was assessing herself accurately and that Peter was overreacting. Vicky was not being carried away by her feelings—not at the moment, at least; if anything she was showing a lot of restraint. Peter *was* treating her like a child.

"Vicky," I said, "perhaps Peter doesn't understand your reasons for wanting to go back to college."

"I admit it might seem like a waste of time," she said. "But that degree means a lot to me. I was devastated when I had to withdraw from college. I felt like a complete failure. Maybe I just need to prove to myself that I can do it. That I'm not . . ." She hesitated before spitting it out: "Not crazy."

Peter was calmer, too. "It's not that we can't afford it," he said. "I just worry that it will be too much for her, that she'll get sick again. And she gets so angry when we talk about it; she seems obsessed with this idea. That's not normal, is it?"

"I don't think trying to decide how much obsessiveness is normal or abnormal is going to help us here, Peter," I said. "It seems to me that the problem is that Vicky is investing a lot of time and emotional energy in a project that you don't think is worthwhile."

"That's right," Peter said decisively.

"But *I* think it's worthwhile," Vicky said. "Just because I have a psychiatric illness doesn't invalidate me as a person. It doesn't mean I need someone to make all my decisions for me."

"Honey, I'm just trying to help you, to protect you—"

Vicky snapped back, "I don't want to be protected, I want to have a real life."

"Wait a minute, wait a minute," I said. "I think we were getting somewhere. Let's go back to Vicky's reasons for wanting to go back to school."

This struggle between Peter and Vicky illustrates a very common problem that can come up in families in which an individual has been diagnosed with a bipolar illness. It's possible to jump to the conclusion that everything the person with the diagnosis does that might be foolish or risky is a symptom of illness, even to the point where the person is hauled into the psychiatrist's office for a "medication adjustment" every time he or she disagrees with spouse, partner, or parents. As with Peter and Vicky, a vicious cycle can get going wherein some bold idea or enthusiasm, or even plain old foolishness or stubbornness, is labeled as "getting manic," leading to feelings of anger and resentment in the person with the diagnosis. When these angry feelings get expressed, they seem to confirm the family's suspicion that the person is "getting sick again," leading to more criticism, more anger, and so on. "He's getting sick again" sometimes becomes a self-fulfilling prophecy: so much anger and emotional stress get generated that a relapse *does* occur because the person with the illness stops taking the medication that controls his or her symptoms, out of frustration and anger and shame: "Why bother staying well, if I'm *always* treated as if I were sick?"

So how does one walk this fine line between not taking every feeling and behavior at face value in a person with bipolar disorder and not invalidating "real" feelings by calling them symptoms? I think communication is the key: honest and open communication. Ask the person with the illness about his or her moods, make observations about behaviors, express concerns in a caring, supportive way. Go along with your family member to doctors' appointments, and share your observations and concerns during the visit in his or her presence. Above all, do not call the therapist or psychiatrist and say, "I don't want my _____ [husband, wife, son, daughter; fill in the blank] to know that I called you, but I think it's important to tell you that. . ." There's nothing more infuriating or demeaning than to have someone sneaking around reporting on you behind your back.

But it's also possible to err on the side of not being involved enough in treatment for fear of being a "tattletale," assuming that the clinicians will notice the same things you've noticed about changes in moods or behaviors. One of the most valuable ways a family member can help is to provide a clear, undistorted view of the situation to the clinical team treating the illness. In my experience, family members are frequently the first to pick up on subtle changes in behaviors and attitudes that signal the beginnings of a relapse. I don't know how many times I have seen patients in the clinic or even in the emergency room who reassured me that they were feeling fine, whose behavior and mood seemed normal, whom I sent on their way with a note in the chart that they were doing well, only to receive a panicked phone call from a spouse or other relative a few hours later: "Didn't she tell you that she's lost ten pounds?" ". . . that he hasn't slept in three nights?" ". . . that he got fired from his job?" Contrary to popular belief, psychiatrists cannot read minds! Become involved with treatment, and communicate your concerns openly, sincerely, and supportively—almost anything that might otherwise seem intrusive can be forgiven.

Remember that your goal is to have your family member trust you when he or she feels most vulnerable and fragile. He or she is already dealing with feelings of deep shame, failure, and loss of control related to having a psychiatric illness. Be supportive, and, yes, be constructively critical when criticism is warranted. But above all, be open, honest, and sincere.

Involuntary Treatment and Other Legal Issues

In every community there are laws and procedures to safeguard individuals who are unable to care for themselves. Laws allowing the removal of children from the care of parents who are abusing them are the most obvious example. Another set of laws are those allowing individuals to be treated for psychiatric illnesses against their will in certain circumstances. One of the most difficult things a person might be called on to do for a family member with bipolar disorder is to initiate involuntary treatment or commitment. But given the power of this illness (especially bipolar I) to cloud judgment and create dangerous situations, there is sometimes no choice but to force the treatment issue in this way. It is always a last resort, but it can literally be lifesaving.

Commitment laws are usually state laws and so vary from one state to another; in addition to these state-by-state variations, local procedures can vary from community to community. This means that I can't provide a step-by-step procedure here, only general principles. But in my experience it's not the procedures that confuse people, it's the general principles, so I think a brief discussion will be worthwhile.

Law and legal procedures governing the provision of psychiatric treatment—or any kind of medical treatment, for that matter—against a persons's stated wishes are based on the knowledge that an individual whose judgment is clouded by the symptoms of an illness often does not make the same decisions about treatment that he or she would make otherwise. The delirious motor vehicle accident victim who has suffered massive blood loss may moan "I want to go home" as he or she loses consciousness on the stretcher, but the ER team will ignore such a statement and proceed to do what they have to do to save the person's life. It is presumed that if the person were alert and thinking clearly and understood the implications of "going home," he or she would not make such a request. Similar principles underlie psychiatric commitment law: treatment is given to persons against their will if clouded judgment prevents them from making good decisions about their treatment. Depressed individuals may be so hopeless that they feel treatment has no chance of helping. Thinking processes in mania can be so disorganized and scattered that seeking out and cooperating with treatment is not possible. In either case there are mechanisms to get needed treatment for persons whose psychiatric symptoms blind them to the need for it.

Fortunately these laws also have safeguards built in to prevent confinement in a psychiatric hospital for the wrong reasons. Decades ago it was very easy to invoke commitment law, and it often required only the signature of a relative or family physician to hospitalize a person for weeks or months, even years. People were hospitalized for all kinds of bogus reasons, and serious abuses of individual rights occurred. Laws became much stricter in the 1960s and 1970s to prevent these abuses. The main change was the addition of *dangerousness* as a commitment criterion. Unless an individual's behavior endangers himself or herself—usually meaning suicidal behavior—or others, the person cannot be committed for involuntary psychiatric treatment.

Requests or petitions for involuntary commitment do not necessarily mean that the person who is alleged to be psychiatrically ill will be hospitalized. Friends and relatives cannot sign a patient in to a hospital; only a doctor can do so. The family's request for involuntary commitment usually will allow the patient to be transported to an emergency room, where a physician will make a decision about hospitalization. The patient may be released if he or she does not meet legal criteria for commitment.

Involuntary commitment is a legal procedure in which an individual is confined against his or her will and temporarily loses some rights of self-determination. For this reason the law and the courts take involuntary psychiatric treatment very seriously, and many safeguards against abuses are built in to the procedures. The person requesting the involuntary commitment must usually appear in person at the local courthouse or police station to give information and, in some jurisdictions, make a sworn statement before a judge or magistrate. Family or friends will be asked for very specific and detailed information about behaviors. This is often frustrating for those trying to get help for their loved one. They may feel that it's uncaring for them to be asked such a lot of questions or that their judgment or motives are being questioned. It's important to remember that in the days when individuals could be confined to psychiatric hospitals simply because a relative or doctor "thought it was best" for them, there were significant abuses of civil rights. When there is serious attention on the part of the issuing magistrate or judge to documenting the facts and close questioning of the need for involuntary treatment, it means that the system is working.

There is a judicial review (a "commitment hearing") at some point (usually a few days after hospitalization) wherein a judge or hearing officer determines that the commitment procedure was done properly and legally. Although this is a legal proceeding, it is not a big courtroom scene. Usually a conference room in the hospital is used, only a few people are present, and the proceedings are kept confidential (they are not a matter of public record). The patient is allowed legal representation; in fact an attorney will be appointed to represent the patient if he or she cannot afford to hire one.

Involuntary commitment for psychiatric treatment does not usually affect a person's other legal rights. Wills or other legal instruments he or she has executed are not invalidated, and patients do not become legally "incompetent" in other areas. Hospitalization and treatment are the only issues that are addressed in commitment hearings.

Occasionally I have seen individuals with severe, poorly controlled bipolar disorder whose families make legal arrangements to safeguard the individuals' financial assets in case another severe episode of the illness comes upon them. This can involve actually having a legally appointed guardian who might control access to bank accounts, prevent the sale of property or other assets, and so forth. Although rarely necessary, this is a valuable option that can go a long way toward preventing financial ruin caused by manic spending sprees. A document called a *power of attorney* can convey certain specific responsibilities and powers—and not others—and does not constitute guardianship. Careful consideration and consultation with an attorney are, of course, necessary so that legally binding documents with safeguards appropriate to the situation can be drafted.

I am aware that the topic of this section of the chapter is a very frightening one, especially to persons with bipolar disorder to whom it might seem that liberty and the right of self-determination can be taken away all too easily. At the risk of sounding glib, however, I want to reassure you that involuntary commitment of an individual is *not* a quick and easy procedure. On the contrary, in my experience most people are surprised at how difficult it is to invoke these laws, how many safeguards are built in to the procedures, and how seriously the strict interpretation of the laws is taken by everyone involved. These laws have been carefully written in the interest of helping, not simply confining, people with severe psychiatric illnesses. In my experience they are effective at doing just that.

More on Safety

Never forget that bipolar disorder can occasionally precipitate truly dangerous behavior. Kay Jamison writes of the "dark, fierce and damaging energy" of mania,[1] and the even darker specter of suicidal violence haunts those with serious depression. Violence is often a difficult subject to deal with because the idea is deeply imbedded in us from an early age that violence is primitive and uncivilized and represents a kind of failure or breakdown in character. Of course we recognize that the person in the grip of psychiatric illness is not violent because of some personal failing, and perhaps because of this there is sometimes a hesitation to admit the need for a proper response to a situation that is getting out of control: when there is some threat of violence, toward either self or others.

I've already talked a bit about suicidal thinking, and it bears repeating that people with bipolar disorder are at much higher risk for suicidal behavior than the general population. Although family members cannot and should not be expected to take the place of psychiatric professionals in evaluating suicide risk, it is important to have some familiarity with the issue. As I've already mentioned, patients who are starting to have suicidal thoughts are often intensely ashamed of them. They will often hint about "feeling desperate," about "not being able to go on," but may not verbalize actual self-destructive thoughts. It's important not to ignore these statements but rather to clarify them. Don't be afraid to ask, "Are you having thoughts of hurting yourself?" People are usually relieved to be able to talk about these feelings and get them out into the open where they can be dealt with. But they may need permission and support in order to do so.

Remember that the period of recovery from a depressive episode can be one of especially high risk for suicidal behavior. People who have been immobilized by depression sometimes develop a higher risk for hurting themselves as they begin to get better and their energy level and ability to act improve. Patients having mixed symptoms—depressed mood and agitated, restless, hyperactive behavior—may also be at higher risk for self-harm. In fact there is some evidence that mixed or dysphoric mania is the most dangerous mood state in this regard.[2]

Another factor that increases risk of suicide is substance abuse, especially alcohol abuse. Alcohol not only worsens mood, it lowers inhibitions. People will do things when drunk that they wouldn't do otherwise. Increased use of alcohol increases the risk of suicidal behaviors and is definitely a worrisome development that needs to be confronted and acted upon.

The development of serious suicidal risk calls for action. Have an emergency plan, and be prepared to use it. Don't hesitate to invoke involuntary commitment procedures if you are really worried and the patient is disputing the need for evaluation.

A less frequent but nevertheless very real risk of violence is the violence toward others that can occur in mania. Friends and family members should not hesitate to call for police help if they feel threatened. "What will the neighbors think?" should not be an issue where safety is concerned. If the situation is becoming dangerous, don't call the psychiatrist's office or the local emergency room; dial 911. Police officers are accustomed to dealing with psychiatrically ill individuals. They know safe physical-restraint techniques, and they will be familiar with psychiatric emergency services in the community. In my experience police officers will have the same goals you will in the situation: transporting the patient quickly and safely to the appropriate health-care facility so that he or she can receive proper treatment.

Getting Support

It's important that family members recognize their own need for support, encouragement, and understanding in dealing with this illness. Mental-health professionals go home every day and leave their work of dealing with psychiatric illnesses behind, an option that family members often do not have. It can be exhausting to live with a hypomanic person and frustrating to deal with a seriously depressed person day after day. The changes and unpredictability of the moods of someone with bipolar disorder intrude into home life and can be the source of severe stress in relationships, straining them to the breaking point.

Perhaps the most difficult challenge is that posed by a family member with bipolar disorder who is resistant to getting treatment. The most astonishing learning experience that medical students and interns have is with their first patient who repeatedly refuses to continue with a treatment that will keep him or her well and out of the hospital. I remember as a resident reading the chart of a bipolar patient who had been admitted to the hospital dozens of times after stopping lithium. Why on earth, I wondered, would a person make such a foolish decision again and again? I remember thinking that taking three capsules of lithium a day seemed a very small inconvenience compared with spending what added to up to several years of this patient's life in a psychiatric hospital. I've since learned that making peace with the illness and with the idea of staying in treatment is much more difficult than healthy people realize (see chapter 20). But the harder lesson is learning that there is no way anyone can *force* a person to take responsibility for his or her treatment. Unless the patient makes the commitment to do so, no amount of love and support, sympathy and understanding, cajoling or even threatening, can make someone take this step. Even family members who understand this at some level may feel guilty, inadequate, and angry at times dealing with this situation. These are very normal feelings. Family members should not be ashamed of these feelings of frustration and anger but rather get help with them.

Even when the patient does take responsibility and is trying to stay well, relapses can occur. Family members might then wonder what *they* did wrong. Did I put too much pressure on? Could I have been more supportive? Why didn't I notice the symptoms coming on sooner and get him or her to the doctor? A hundred questions, a thousand "if only's," another round of guilt, frustration, and anger.

On the other side of this issue is another set of questions: How much understanding and support for the bipolar person might be too much? What is protective, and what is overprotective? Should you call your loved one's boss with excuses as to why he or she isn't at work? Should you pay off credit card debts from hypomanic spending sprees caused by dropping out of treatment? What actions constitute helping a sick person, and what actions are helping a person to be sick? These are thorny, complex questions that have no easy answers.

For all these reasons it's vital that family members go along with the patient to support groups—and go to support groups themselves even if the patient will not go—and consider getting counseling or therapy for themselves to deal with the stresses caused by this illness. Comprehensive programs for the treatment of persons with bipolar disorder are increasingly emphasizing family involvement.

Like many chronic illnesses, bipolar disorder afflicts one but affects many in the family. It's important that *all* those affected get the help, support, and encouragement they need.

CHAPTER 23

Looking Ahead

SEVERAL YEARS AGO I READ IN A MAGAZINE ARTICLE THAT SCIENTISTS know more about outer space than they do about the human brain. Fortunately that is changing very, very rapidly. We know vastly more about brain function now than we did only a few years ago, and the pace of new discoveries is accelerating. One of the main reasons for this acceleration is the availability of new tools with which to do research.

Thanks to the development of sophisticated biochemical techniques, we are learning more and more about what goes on *inside* the neuron, discovering the details of the workings of these fantastic living computers. With the discovery of G proteins and with the realization that this is probably where lithium works to bring about its therapeutic effect, we move ever closer to identifying exactly what is "broken" in bipolar disorder. As we do, we shall be able to develop new and better pharmaceuticals that can be *designed* for the job they need to do, not discovered accidentally, as lithium and valproate were.

New technologies for brain imaging such as PET and a related technique called SPECT (for "single photon emission computed tomography") are allowing scientists to see the brain at work in living persons for the first time. These imaging techniques can show changes in blood flow within the brain, locate areas that are hyperactive or abnormally low in activity, or detect abnormally high or abnormally low levels of brain chemicals like serotonin and dopamine. This information is revealing that the interplay of activity between different brain areas is important in the regulation of mood and is allowing the identification of the circuitry responsible. These techniques are allowing us to see how the brain of the person with the mood disorder functions differently from that of a person who does not have a mood disorder, and, perhaps even more interesting, what changes occur when a person receives treatment and is beginning to feel well again.

Perhaps the most exciting work is being done in the field of genetics. Here again it is the development of new biochemical methods and molecular probes that is making this research possible. The discovery of new genes is announced every day, and it is only a matter of time before the genetic mechanisms of bipolar disorder are unraveled. But the identification of genes responsible for mood disorders is only one of the goals of work in this field. Just as important will be understanding the mechanisms by which genes turn on and off and other mechanisms that regulate the expression and work of the instructions encoded in the DNA molecule.

Advances in many seemingly unrelated fields hold promise for better understanding of bipolar disorder too—advances in computer technology, for example. Just as architects now use computers to visualize buildings before they are built, pharmacologists are working to design new drugs by using computers to visualize the three-dimensional structures of neurotransmitters, receptors, and possible pharmaceutical agents. It is hoped that new pharmaceuticals that have a better "fit" at their active site will work faster, at lower doses, and with fewer side effects. Computers are also being used to model and study brain activity. Remember that the brain is much more than just a sophisticated computer; it is more like a network of millions and millions of individual computers. Advanced computers using *nonsequential neural architecture* to build *neural networks*—made up of many interconnected but independently computing units—show properties that would not be predicted from known principles of computing. These properties are probably highly relevant to the study of human brain activity and psychiatric illness. One researcher has even proposed a computer model for the manic state using this type of computer network model.[1]

Our understanding of the biology of mood disorders is getting better all the time. With each advance we get closer to better diagnostic methods and safer and more effective treatments. The number of new medications continues to grow, and many more new pharmaceuticals are "in the pipeline." More sophisticated use of nonpharmaceutical treatments like sleep phase advance and phototherapy may make it possible to use lower doses of medications or may help medications to work more quickly. We are just beginning to learn how to use transcranial magnetic stimulation to treat mood disorders. If this novel treatment is as effective as it is safe, it may represent the greatest breakthrough in the treatment of psychiatric disorders since the discovery of the therapeutic effects of lithium in the 1940s.

The research into the genetics of bipolar disorder promises great breakthroughs in the diagnosis and treatment of mood disorders. Not only will this work improve our ability to diagnose bipolar disorder, it may lead to treatment breakthroughs as well. If we can make the step from isolating genes to determining the function of those genes, we shall be able to design treatments more effectively and more rationally. This work also holds out the possibility of gene therapy: repairing the code in the DNA that causes bipolar disorder. The obstacles to be overcome before we dare look for this type of cure can only be called daunting, even monumental. But scientists are closing in on bipolar disorder little by little, and with enough time and enough hard work, a cure might be possible.

Patients frequently ask me if they will have to take medication for the rest of their lives. I always tell them that no one knows the answer to that question because no one knows exactly what the treatment of bipolar disorder might be in the future. Physicians practicing in the 1930s probably could not imagine that vaccines would practically eliminate diphtheria, polio, measles, and the other childhood diseases they saw so much of but were completely helpless to treat. The astonishing developments in neuroscience and genetics hold just as much promise for sufferers of bipolar disorder.

There is much reason to hope for great strides in our ability to diagnose and effectively treat this illness. But we have *already* made great strides; individuals with bipolar disorder must not let denial or fear stand in the way of taking advantage of the very good treatments that we have available. Ignorance is no excuse, either. Organizations such as the National Depressive and Manic-Depressive Association provide up-to-date information about bipolar disorder in newsletters, in brochures, and, most important, in the support groups they sponsor. With the development of the Internet and ever growing on-line resources, anyone with access to a computer can get the very latest information on new pharmaceuticals and other treatments with the click of a computer mouse.

Like many serious illnesses, bipolar disorder can be life-threatening. Unlike some others, however, it has a unique capacity to rob individuals of their spirit, to take over their humanity. And yet some of its sufferers have taken inspiration from their struggle with this illness and have produced works of art and music and literature that have inspired and exhilarated the world. Millions of others are simply living with bipolar disorder but taking charge, learning about the illness and, yes, learning *from* the illness about themselves, about what it means to be human.

Resources

SUGGESTED READING

Goodwin, Frederick K., and Kay Redfield Jamison. *Manic-Depressive Illness.* New York: Oxford University Press, 1990.
> An encyclopedic work for scientists and clinicians—comprehensive, but definitely "industrial-strength" reading. A superb reference book.

Jamison, Kay Redfield. *Touched with Fire: Manic-Depressive Illness and the Artistic Temperament.* New York: Free Press, 1993.
> A thorough survey of creative individuals who suffered from bipolar disorder, and an excellent discussion of the connections between creativity and mood disorders.

Jamison, Kay Redfield. *An Unquiet Mind: A Memoir of Moods and Madness.* New York: Vintage Books, 1996.
> A powerful and moving narrative written with grace and wit by an international expert on the illness who suffers from it herself. This treasure of a book contains some of the most engrossing and vivid descriptions of the experience of bipolar disorder ever written. A "must read" for anyone touched by bipolar disorder.

Kraepelin, Emil. *Manic-Depressive Insanity and Paranoia.* Trans. R. M. Barclay, ed. G. M. Robertson. 1921; reprint, New York: Arno Press, 1976.
> Many college and university libraries have a copy of this book. Arguably the very first textbook on the illness ever written, it is definitely worth reading.

Rosenthal, Norman E. *Winter Blues: Seasonal Affective Disorder, What It Is and How to Overcome It.* New York: Guilford Press, 1993.

> A comprehensive and highly readable discussion of seasonal affective disorder.

Styron, William. *Darkness Visible: A Memoir of Madness.* New York: Random House, 1990.

> I recommend this book to medical students as one of the best accounts of the symptoms of depression available. A good book for family members to read to better understand the experience of serious depression.

SUPPORT AND ADVOCACY ORGANIZATIONS

All of the following organizations provide information and resources, and many offer referrals to support groups as well as to clinicians in your community who are skilled in treating mood disorders. Contact them all and become a member! In addition to the direct services they provide to consumers, they are active in combating the stigmatization of psychiatric illnesses, in lobbying for better medical insurance coverage for psychiatric disorders, and in supporting research.

The Depression and Related Affective Disorders Association (DRADA)
Meyer 3-181, 550 Building
Johns Hopkins Hospital
600 North Wolfe Street
Baltimore, MD 21287-7381
410-955-4647
http://infonet.welch.jhu.edu/departments/drada/default

National Alliance for the Mentally Ill (NAMI)
200 N. Glebe Road, Suite 1015
Arlington, VA 22203-3754
800-950-6264
http://www.nami.org

The National Depressive and Manic-Depressive Association (NDMDA)
730 North Franklin Street
Chicago, IL 60610
800-82-NDMDA
http://www.ndmda.org

The National Foundation for Depressive Illness, Inc.
P.O. Box 2257
New York, NY 10116
800-239-1265
http://www.depression.org

National Mental Health Association (NMHA)
1021 Prince Street
Alexandria, VA 22314
800-969-NMHA
http://www.nmha.org

All of the support and advocacy groups listed in the previous section have sites on the World Wide Web, and the astonishing range of resources on the Internet continues to grow. Remember, however, that there are also inaccurate information, bias, and just plain nonsense on the Internet, and that it's important to consider information sources very carefully.

Here are some excellent resources:

The American Psychiatric Press, Inc.
http://www.appi.org
> Access to several of the most important and influential professional publications for psychiatrists: the *American Journal of Psychiatry,* the *Journal of Neuropsychiatry and Clinical Neurosciences,* and others (scientific publications written for physicians and scientists).

The Harvard Mental Health Letter
http://www.med.harvard.edu/publications/Health_Publications/mntlns.html
> This is the on-line edition of a popular newsletter written mostly for professionals but in a style that's usually easily understood by informed lay persons. Up-to-date news from an authoritative source.

Internet Mental Health
http://www.mentalhealth.com
> An excellent site with information on many different disorders and their treatments, information on many psychiatric medications, and hundreds of reference articles from popular and professional publications.

Medscape
http://www.medscape.com
> This is primarily a news site for medical professionals, but it also has a "patient information" section with many useful articles and links to other resources.

Moodswing.org
http://www.moodswing.org
> Many resources on bipolar disorder, including reading materials, an "FAQ" (frequently asked questions) section on bipolar disorder, and links to many other sources.

Pendulum Resources
http://www.pendulum.org
> Another storehouse of information on bipolar disorder with an on-line bookstore and links to other useful sites.

Support Group.com
http://www.support-group.com

> Dozens of pages on different disorders, including several on bipolar disorder. Bulletin boards and "chats" for patients, for significant others, and "Bipolar Teens." Well-organized and, judging from the number of people leaving messages, a popular and useful resource for a lot of people.

United States National Library of Medicine
http://www.nlm.nih.gov

> This site provides free access to Medline, the most comprehensive medical database in the world. Over eight million references in thirty-eight hundred journals can be accessed. An incredibly valuable resource!

The following Internet newsgroups will be of interest to people with bipolar disorder:

alt.support.depression.manic
soc.support.depression.family
soc.support.depression.manic

Notes

PREFACE

1. For a discussion of the diagnosis of bipolar disorder in these historical person-
alities, see Kay Redfield Jamison, *Touched with Fire: Manic-Depressive Illness and the
Artistic Temperament* (New York: Free Press, 1993).

2. Gabor Keitner, Ivan Miller, M. Tracie Shea, and Martin Keller, "Course of Illness and Maintenance Treatments for Patients with Bipolar Disorder," *Journal of Clinical Psychiatry* 56, no. 1 (1995): 5–13.

3. "National Survey of NDMDA Members Finds Long Delay in Diagnosis of
Manic-Depressive Illness," in "News and Notes," *Hospital and Community Psychiatry*
44, no. 8 (1993): 800–801.

4. Frederick K. Goodwin and Kay Redfield Jamison, *Manic-Depressive Illness*
(New York: Oxford University Press, 1990), 228.

CHAPTER 1. NORMAL AND ABNORMAL MOOD

1. *Webster's Ninth New Collegiate Dictionary,* ed. Frederick C. Mish (Springfield,
Mass.: Merriam-Webster, 1984).

2. Although I have made these clinical vignettes as realistic as possible by using
symptom details culled from many patients, they are fictitious and do not portray any
person living or dead.

3. The word *mania* has very ancient origins, deriving from the Greek word
mainesthai, which means simply "to be insane." Very early English physicians sometimes used the word *madness* to describe the syndrome of disorganized hyperactivity
that we now call mania. But during the eighteenth and nineteenth centuries, European
physicians writing about mental disorders increasingly used the term *mania* (in French

la manie and in German *die Manie*). When Emil Kraepelin used the term *manic-depressive insanity* in his ground-breaking work on bipolar disorder, the use of the term *mania* for the excited phase of the disorder became firmly established.

4. Henry J. Berkley, *A Treatise on Mental Diseases* (1900; reprint, New York: Arno Press, 1980), 143.

5. Kay Redfield Jamison, *An Unquiet Mind: A Memoir of Moods and Madness* (New York: Vintage Books, 1996), 36.

6. Frederick K. Goodwin and Kay Redfield Jamison, *Manic-Depressive Illness* (New York: Oxford University Press, 1990), 23.

7. Quoted in ibid., 26–27.

8. Emil Kraepelin, *Manic-Depressive Insanity and Paranoia*, trans. R. M. Barclay, ed. G. M. Robertson (1921; reprint, New York: Arno Press, 1976), 31. This is a translation of volumes 3 and 4 of the eighth edition (1913) of Kraepelin's textbook *Psychiatrie*, which originally appeared in 1896.

9. Goodwin and Jamison, *Manic-Depressive Illness*, 29.

10. Kraepelin, *Manic-Depressive Insanity*, 31.

11. For a discussion of the concept of motivated behaviors in psychiatry, see Paul McHugh and Philip Slavney, *The Perspectives of Psychiatry* (Baltimore: Johns Hopkins University Press, 1986), 105–7.

12. Kraepelin, *Manic-Depressive Insanity*, 62.

13. Ibid., 56, 64.

14. J. D. Campbell, *Manic-Depressive Disease: Clinical and Psychiatric Significance* (Philadelphia: J. D. Lippincott, 1953), 159–60, quoted in Goodwin and Jamison, *Manic-Depressive Illness*, 24.

15. Jamison, *Unquiet Mind*, 83.

16. Kraepelin, *Manic-Depressive Insanity*, 70.

17. Berkley, *Treatise on Mental Diseases*, 160.

18. Gabrielle Carlson and Frederick Goodwin, "The Stages of Mania," *Archives of General Psychiatry* 28 (1973): 221–28.

19. Quoted in Edward Hare, "The Two Manias: Study of the Evolution of the Modern Concept of Mania," *British Journal of Psychiatry* 138 (1981): 89–99.

20. Norman Endler, *Holiday of Darkness: A Psychologist's Personal Journey out of His Depression* (New York: John Wiley and Sons, 1982), 4.

21. Ibid., 86.

22. William Styron, *Darkness Visible: A Memoir of Madness* (New York: Random House, 1990), 19.

23. Endler, *Holiday of Darkness*, 48–49.

24. Johann Wolfgang von Goethe, *The Sorrows of Young Werther*, trans. Elizabeth Mayer and Louise Bogan (New York: Random House, 1971), 114.

25. Quoted in Kay Redfield Jamison, *Touched with Fire: Manic-Depressive Illness and the Artistic Temperament* (New York: Free Press, 1993), 21.

26. Styron, *Darkness Visible*, 17.

27. Endler, *Holiday of Darkness*, 29.

28. Kraepelin, *Manic-Depressive Insanity*, 75.

29. F. Scott Fitzgerald, *The Crackup* (New York: New Directions, 1956), 75.

30. Styron, *Darkness Visible,* 17.

31. Endler, *Holiday of Darkness,* 54.

32. Styron, *Darkness Visible,* 44.

33. Endler, *Holiday of Darkness,* 46.

34. Kraepelin, *Manic-Depressive Insanity,* 84.

35. Ibid., 89.

36. Styron, *Darkness Visible,* 58.

37. Kraepelin, *Manic-Depressive Insanity,* 97.

38. Jamison, *Unquiet Mind,* 45.

39. Dr. Claude Brouchier, 1679, quoted in Goodwin and Jamison, *Manic-Depressive Illness,* 45.

40. Kraepelin, *Manic-Depressive Insanity,* 105–6.

41. Ibid., 104.

42. See Susan McElroy, Paul Keck, Harrison Pope, James Hudson, Giannni Faedda, and Alan Swann, "Clinical and Research Implications of the Diagnosis of Dysphoric or Mixed Mania or Hypomania," *American Journal of Psychiatry* 149 (1992): 1633–44.

43. Kraepelin, *Manic-Depressive Insanity,* 99.

CHAPTER 2. THE DIAGNOSIS OF BIPOLAR DISORDER

Epigraph: Emil Kraepelin, *Manic-Depressive Insanity and Paranoia,* trans. R. M. Barclay, ed. G. M. Robertson (1921; reprint, New York: Arno Press, 1976), 193.

1. Frederick K. Goodwin and Kay Redfield Jamison, *Manic-Depressive Illness* (New York: Oxford University Press, 1990), 132.

2. Modern diagnostic classifications are usually different from those that were used when these older studies were done. In most cases, however, patients with "manic-depressive illness" in these studies had full-blown manic episodes and severe depressions and thus would today probably be diagnosed with bipolar I. Nevertheless, cases that would today be diagnosed differently (as bipolar II, for example) may have been mixed in. Thus, the findings and statistics must be interpreted with some caution.

3. Thomas A. C. Rennie, "Prognosis in Manic-Depressive Psychosis," *American Journal of Psychiatry* 98 (1942): 801–14, quoted in Goodwin and Jamison, *Manic-Depressive Illness,* 133.

4. Kraepelin, *Manic-Depressive Insanity,* 136.

5. Ibid., 3, 137.

6. G. Winokur, P. Clayton, and T. Reich, *Manic-Depressive Illness* (St. Louis: C. V. Mosby, 1969), quoted in Goodwin and Jamison, *Manic-Depressive Illness,* 141.

7. Athansio Koukopoulas, Daniela Reginaldi, Giampolo Minnai, Gino Serre, Luca Pani, and Neil Johnson, "The Long Term Prophylaxis of Affective Disorders," in *Depression and Mania: From Neurobiology to Treatment,* ed. G. Gessa, W. Fratta, L. Pina, and G. Serre (New York: Raven Press, 1995), 127–47.

8. William Coryell, Nancy Andreasen, Jean Endicott, and Martin Keller, "The Significance of Past Mania or Hypomania in the Course and Outcome of Major Depression," *American Journal of Psychiatry* 144 (1987): 309–15.

9. G. Cassano, H. Akiskal, M. Savina, L. Musetti, and G. Perugi, "Proposed Subtypes of Bipolar II and Related Disorders: With Hypomanic Episodes (or Cyclothymia) and with Hyperthymic Temperament," *Journal of Affective Disorders* 26 (1992): 127–40.

10. See Sylvia Simpson, Susan Folstein, Deborah Meyers, Francis McMahon, Diane Brusco, and J. Raymond DePaulo, "Bipolar II: The Most Common Bipolar Phenotype?" *American Journal of Psychiatry* 150 (1993): 901–3.

11. Hagop Akiskal, Jack Maser, Pamela Zeller, Jean Endicott, William Coryell, Martin Keller, Meredith Warshaw, Paula Clayton, and Frederick Goodwin, "Switching from 'Unipolar' to Bipolar II: An Eleven-Year Prospective Study of Clinical and Temperamental Predictors in 559 Patients," *Archives of General Psychiatry* 52 (1995): 114–23.

12. Goodwin and Jamison, *Manic-Depressive Illness*, 69.

13. Simpson, Folstein, Meyers, McMahon, Brusco, and DePaulo, "Bipolar II: The Most Common Bipolar Phenotype?"

14. Kraepelin, *Manic-Depressive Insanity*, 131.

15. Hagop S. Akiskal, "The Prevalent Clinical Spectrum of Bipolar Disorders: Beyond DSM-IV," *Journal of Clinical Psychopharmacology* 16, suppl. (1996): 4S–14S.

16. Kraepelin, *Manic-Depressive Insanity*, 132.

17. H. Akiskal, M. K. Khani, and A. Scott-Strauss, "Cyclothymic Temperamental Disorders," *Psychiatric Clinics of North America* 2 (1979): 527–54.

18. Robert Howland and Michael Thase, "A Comprehensive Review of Cyclothymic Disorder," *Journal of Nervous and Mental Disease* 181 (1993): 485–93.

19. Akiskal, "Prevalent Clinical Spectrum of Bipolar Disorders."

20. Howland and Thase, "Comprehensive Review of Cyclothymic Disorder," 485–93.

21. Kraepelin, *Manic-Depressive Insanity*, 2.

22. Hagop Akiskal and Gopinath Mallya, "Criteria for 'Soft' Bipolar Spectrum: Treatment Implications," *Psychopharmacology Bulletin* 23, no. 1 (1987): 68–73.

23. Akiskal, "Prevalent Clinical Spectrum of Bipolar Disorders."

24. American Psychiatric Association, *Diagnostic and Statistical Manual of Mental Disorders,* 4th ed. (Washington, D.C.: American Psychiatric Association, 1994), 390–91.

25. See Goodwin and Jamison, *Manic-Depressive Illness*, 136–38.

26. R. W. Cowdry, T. A. Wehr, A. Zis, and F. K. Goodwin, "Thyroid Abnormalities Associated with Rapid Cycling Bipolar Illness," *Archives of General Psychiatry* 40 (1983): 414–20, and T. A. Wehr and F. K. Goodwin, "Rapid Cycling in Manic-Depressives Induced by Tricyclic Antidepressants," *Archives of General Psychiatry* 36 (1979): 555–59.

27. A. Koukopoulas, B. Caliari, A. Tundo, G. Floris, D. Reginaldi, and L. Tondo, "Rapid Cyclers, Temperament, and Antidepressants," *Comprehensive Psychiatry* 24, no. 3 (1983): 249–58.

28. William Coryell, Jean Endicott, and Martin Keller, "Rapid Cycling Bipolar Disorder: Demographics, Diagnosis, Family History, and Course," *Archives of General Psychiatry* 49 (1992): 126–31.

CHAPTER 3. A SUMMARY OF THE DIAGNOSTIC CATEGORIES
OF BIPOLAR DISORDER IN *DSM IV*

1. American Psychiatric Association, *Diagnostic and Statistical Manual of Mental Disorders,* 4th ed. (Washington, D.C.: American Psychiatric Association, 1994), xvii. Note that "epilepsy" was at the time considered to be a mental illness.

2. Alfred Kinsey, Wardell Pomeroy, and Clyde Martin, *Sexual Behavior in the Human Male* (Philadelphia: W. B. Saunders, 1948), 678, 639.

CHAPTER 4. THE MOOD DISEASE

1. Quoted in Stanley W. Jackson, *Melancholia and Depression, from Hippocratic Times to Modern Times* (New Haven: Yale University Press, 1986), 251 ("peevish," "complain[ed]," "At the height"), and in Frederick K. Goodwin and Kay Redfield Jamison, *Manic-Depressive Illness* (New York: Oxford University Press, 1990), 58 ("in my opinion").

2. Quoted in Jackson, *Melancholia and Depression,* 253–54.

3. Quoted in ibid., 257.

4. See ibid., 262–63.

5. Emil Kraepelin, *Manic-Depressive Insanity and Paranoia,* trans. R. M. Barclay, ed. G. M. Robertson (1921; reprint, New York: Arno Press, 1976), 1.

6. Jackson, *Melancholia and Depression,* 272.

7. Henry J. Berkley, *A Treatise on Mental Disorders* (1900; reprint, New York: Arno Press, 1980), 179.

8. John F. J. Cade, "Lithium Salts in the Treatment of Psychotic Excitement," *Medical Journal of Australia* 36 (1949): 349–52.

9. Ibid., 350–51.

10. For a superb account of this shameful story, see Götz Aly, Peter Chroust, and Christian Pross, *Cleansing the Fatherland: Nazi Medicine and Racial Hygiene* (Baltimore: Johns Hopkins University Press, 1994).

11. Ronald R. Fieve, *Moodswing: The Third Revolution in Psychiatry* (New York: Bantam Books, 1975), 3.

12. M. Schou, N. Juel-Nielsen, E. Strömgren, and H. Voldby, "The Treatment of Manic Psychoses by the Administration of Lithium Salts," *Journal of Neurology, Neurosurgery, and Psychiatry* 17 (1954): 250–60.

13. Roland Kuhn, "The Treatment of Depressive States with G 22355 (Imipramine Hydrochloride)," *American Journal of Psychiatry* 115 (1958): 459–64, at 461.

14. Schou, Juel-Nielsen, Strömgren, and Voldby, "Treatment of Manic Psychoses by the Administration of Lithium Salts," 256. Emphasis added.

CHAPTER 5. THE BRAIN: NEURONS, NEUROTRANSMITTERS,
AND MORE

1. Nancy C. Andreason, *The Broken Brain: The Biological Revolution in Psychiatry* (New York: Harper and Row, 1985).

CHAPTER 6. MOOD-STABILIZING MEDICATIONS

1. Anastase Georgotas and Samuel Gershon, "Historical Perspectives and Current Highlights on Lithium Treatment in Manic-Depressive Illness," *Journal of Clinical Psychopharmacology* 1, no. 1 (1981): 27–31.

2. Paul Baalstrup and Morgans Schou, "Lithium as a Prophylactic Agent: Its Effect against Recurrent Depressions and Manic-Depressive Psychosis," *Archives of General Psychiatry* 16, no. 2 (1967): 162–72.

3. B. Blackwell and M. Shephard, "Prophylactic Lithium: Another Therapeutic Myth?" *Lancet* 1 (1968): 968–71.

4. P. Baalstrup, J. Poulsen, M. Schou, K. Thomsen, and A. Amdisen, "Prophylactic Lithium: Double-Blind Discontinuation in Manic and Recurrent-Depressive Disorders," *Lancet* 2 (1970): 326–30.

5. American Psychiatric Association, "Practice Guidelines for the Treatment of Bipolar Disorder," *American Journal of Psychiatry* 151, suppl. (1994): 6.

6. To be more precise, the therapeutic index is the ratio of the largest dose producing no toxic symptoms to the smallest dose routinely producing the desired therapeutic effects.

7. Alan Gelenberg, John Kane, Martin Keller, Phillip Lavori, Jerrold Rosenbaum, Karyl Cole, and Janet Lavelle, "Comparison of Standard and Low Levels of Lithium for Maintenance Treatment of Bipolar Disorder," *New England Journal of Medicine* 321, no. 22 (1989): 1489–93.

8. Morgans Schou, "Forty Years of Lithium Treatment," *Archives of General Psychiatry* 54 (1997): 9–13.

9. Ibid., 11.

10. American Psychiatric Association, "Practice Guidelines for the Treatment of Bipolar Disorder," 7.

11. Frederick K. Goodwin and Kay Redfield Jamison, *Manic-Depressive Illness* (New York: Oxford University Press, 1990), 707.

12. See Charles Bowden and Susan McElroy, "History of the Development of Valproate for the Treatment of Bipolar Disorder," *Journal of Clinical Psychiatry* 56, suppl. 3 (1995): 3–5.

13. American Psychiatric Association, "Practice Guidelines for the Treatment of Bipolar Disorder," 9.

14. Paul Keck, Azmi Nabulsi, Jennifer Taylor, Curtis Henke, Joseph Chmiel, Sean Stanton, and Jerry Bennett, "A Pharmaco-economic Model of Divalproex versus Lithium in the Acute and Prophylactic Treatment of Bipolar I Disorder," *Journal of Clinical Psychiatry* 57, no. 5 (1996): 213–22.

15. Susan McElroy, Paul Keck, Karen Tugrul, and Jerry Bennett, "Valproate as a Loading Treatment in Acute Mania," *Neuropsychobiology* 27 (1993): 146–49.

16. Charles L. Bowden, "Predictors of Response to Divalproex and Lithium," *Journal of Clinical Psychiatry* 56, suppl. 3 (1995): 25–29.

17. Susan McElroy, Paul Keck, Harrison Pope, and James Hudson, "Valproate in Psychiatric Disorders: Literature Review and Clinical Guidelines," *Journal of Clinical Psychiatry* 50, suppl. 3 (1989): 23–29.

18. American Psychiatric Association, "Practice Guidelines for the Treatment of Bipolar Disorder," 21. See also Alan Swann, Charles Bowden, David Morris, Joseph Calabrese, Frederick Petty, Joyce Small, Steven Dilsaver, and John Davis, "Depression during Mania: Treatment Response to Lithium or Divalproex," *Archives of General Psychiatry* 54 (1997): 37–42.

19. American Psychiatric Association, "Practice Guidelines for the Treatment of Bipolar Disorder," 10.

20. See Frederick Jacobsen, "Low-Dose Valproate: A New Treatment for Cyclothymia, Mild Rapid-Cycling Disorders, and Premenstrual Syndrome," *Journal of Clinical Psychiatry* 54, no. 6 (1993): 229–34. Also J. A. Delito, "The Effect of Valproate on Bipolar Spectrum Temperamental Disorders," *Journal of Clinical Psychiatry* 54, no. 8 (1993): 300–304.

21. Gary Sachs, "Bipolar Mood Disorder: Practical Strategies for Acute and Maintenance Phase Treatment," *Journal of Clinical Psychopharmacology* 16, no. 2, suppl. 1 (1996): 32S–47S.

22. J. C. Ballenger and R. M. Post, "Carbamazepine in Manic-Depressive Illness: A New Treatment," *American Journal of Psychiatry* 37 (1980): 782–90.

23. B. Lerer, M. Moore, E. Meyendorff, S. R. Cho, and S. Gershon, "Carbamazepine versus Lithium in Mania: A Double Blind Study," *Journal of Clinical Psychiatry* 48 (1987): 89–93.

24. Robert Post, Thomas Uhde, James Ballenger, and Kathleen Squillace, "Prophylactic Efficacy of Carbamazepine in Manic-Depressive Illness," *American Journal of Psychiatry* 140 (1983): 1602–4.

25. Jonathan Sporn and Gary Sachs, "The Anticonvulsant Lamotrigine in Treatment Resistant Manic-Depressive Illness," *Journal of Clinical Psychopharmacology* 17 (1997): 185–89.

26. Joseph Calabrese, S. Hossein Fatemi, and Mark Woyshville, "Antidepressant Effects of Lamotrigine in Rapid Cycling Bipolar Disorder," *American Journal of Psychiatry* 153 (1996): 1236.

27. Sporn and Sachs, "Anticonvulsant Lamotrigine in Treatment Resistant Manic-Depressive Illness."

28. Sean Stanton, Paul Keck, and Susan McElroy, "Treatment of Acute Mania with Gabapentin," *American Journal of Psychiatry* 154 (1997): 287.

29. Charles Schaffer and Linda Schaffer, Gabapentin in the Treatment of Bipolar Disorder," *American Journal of Psychiatry* 154 (1997): 291.

CHAPTER 7. ANTIDEPRESSANT MEDICATIONS

1. H. S. Lee, D. H. Song, C. H. Kim, and H. K. Choi, "An Open Trial of Fluoxetine in the Treatment of Premature Ejaculation," *Journal of Clinical Psychopharmacology* 16, no. 5 (1993): 379–82.

2. Frederick K. Goodwin and Kay Redfield Jamison, *Manic-Depressive Illness* (New York: Oxford University Press, 1990), 650.

3. Andrew Stoll, Pierre Mayer, Meredith Kolbrener, Eric Goldstein, Barbara Suplit, Judith Lucier, Bruce Cohen, and Mauricio Tohen, "Antidepressant-Associated Mania: A Controlled Comparison with Spontaneous Mania," *American Journal of Psychiatry* 151 (1994): 1642–45. See also Murial Young, Cornelius Pitts, Rosemary Oakes, and Iven Gergel, "A Double-Blind Placebo Controlled Trial Comparing the Effect of Paroxetine and Imipramine in the Treatment of Bipolar Depression," poster #66 presented at the Second International Conference on Bipolar Disorder, sponsored by the

University of Pittsburgh School of Medicine, Center for Continuing Education in the Health Sciences, Pittsburgh, June 19, 1997.

CHAPTER 8. ANTIPSYCHOTIC MEDICATIONS

1. American Psychiatric Association, "Practice Guidelines for the Treatment of Patients with Bipolar Disorder," *American Journal of Psychiatry* 151, suppl. (1994): 12–13.

2. Jeffrey Lieberman, Allan Safferman, Simcha Pollack, Sally Szmanski, Celeste Johns, Alfreda Howard, Michael Kronig, Peter Bookstein, and John Kane, "Clinical Effects of Clozapine in Chronic Schizophrenia: Response to Treatment and Predictors of Outcome," *American Journal of Psychiatry* 151 (1994): 1744–52.

3. In a study of 11,555 patients treated with clozapine, 73, or 0.91 percent, developed agranulocytosis (of whom 2 died of the infectious complications of the condition). See Jose Alvir, Jeffrey Lieberman, Allan Safferman, Jeffrey Schwimmer, and John Schaaf, "Clozapine-Induced Agranulocytosis: Incidence and Risk Factors in the United States," *New England Journal of Medicine* 329 (1993): 162–67.

4. Joseph Calabrese, Herbert Meltzer, and Paul Markovitz, "Clozapine Prophylaxis in Rapid Cycling Bipolar Disorder," *Journal of Clinical Psychopharmacology* 11 (1991): 396–97.

5. Joseph Calabrese, Susan Kimmel, Mark Woyshville, Daniel Rapport, Carl Faust, Paul Thompson, and Herbert Meltzer, "Clozapine for Treatment-Refractory Mania," *American Journal of Psychiatry* 153 (1996): 759–64.

6. Carlos Zarate, Mauricio Tohen, Michael Banov, Michelle Weiss, and Jonathan Cole, "Is Clozapine a Mood Stabilizer?" *Journal of Clinical Psychiatry* 56, no. 3 (1995): 108–12.

7. Mauricio Tohen, Todd Sanger, Gary Tollefson, and Susan McElroy, "Olanzapine versus Haloperidol in the Treatment of Schizoaffective Bipolar Patients," poster #86 presented at the Second International Conference on Bipolar Disorder, sponsored by the University of Pittsburgh School of Medicine, Center for Continuing Education in the Health Sciences, Pittsburgh, June 19, 1997.

CHAPTER 9. OTHER MEDICATIONS, HORMONES, AND AN HERB

1. S. Dubovsky, R. Franks, and M. Lifschitz, "Effectiveness of Verapamil in the Treatment of a Manic Patient," *American Journal of Psychiatry* 139 (1982): 502–3.

2. For an overview of these studies, see Steven Dubovsky and Randall Buzan, "Novel Alternatives and Supplements to Lithium and Anticonvulsants for Bipolar Affective Disorder," *Journal of Clinical Psychiatry* 58 (1997): 224–42.

3. See, for example, Kishore Gadde and K. Ranga Rama Krishman, "Recent Advances in the Pharmacologic Treatment of Bipolar Illness," *Psychiatric Annals* 27 (1997): 496–506.

4. American Psychiatric Association, "Practice Guidelines for the Treatment of Patients with Bipolar Disorder," *American Journal of Psychiatry* 151, suppl. (1994): 14.

5. See the section on the use of "stimulants and euphoriants" in the treatment of acute bipolar depression in Frederick K. Goodwin and Kay Redfield Jamison, *Manic-*

Depressive Illness (New York: Oxford University Press, 1990), 652, for a discussion and list of references on trials of psychostimulants in various depressive disorders. See also P. S. Masand, P. Pickett, and G. B. Murry, "Psychostimulants for Secondary Depression in Medical Illness," *Psychosomatics* 32 (1991): 203–8.

6. American Psychiatric Association, "Practice Guidelines for the Treatment of Patients with Bipolar Disorder," 14.

7. See M. Peet and S. Peters, "Drug Induced Mania," *Drug Safety* 12 (1995): 146–53, and P. S. Masand, P. Pickett, and G. B. Murry, "Hypomania Precipitated by Psychostimulant Use in Depressed Medically Ill Patients," *Psychosomatics* 36 (1995): 145–47.

8. Barbara Bartlik, Peter Kaplan, James Kocsis, Carol Roeloffs, Richard Friedman, and Alan Cohen, "Stimulants for SSRIs-Induced Sexual Dysfunction," poster presented at the 149th Annual Meeting of the American Psychiatric Association, May 4–6, 1996 (NR644).

9. M. S. Bauer, C. Whybrow, and A. Winokur, "Rapid Cycling Bipolar Affective Disorder I: Association with Grade I Hypothyroidism," *Archives of General Psychiatry* 47 (1990): 427–32.

10. H. A. Oomen, A. J. Schipperijn, and H. A. Drexhage, "The Prevalence of Affective Disorder and in Particular of a Rapid Cycling Bipolar Disorder in Patients with Abnormal Thyroid Function Tests," *Clinical Endocrinology* 45 (1996): 215–23.

11. Joseph Calabrese and Mark Woyshville, "A Medication Algorithm for Treatment of Bipolar Rapid Cycling?" *Journal of Clinical Psychiatry* 56, suppl. 3 (1995): 11–18.

12. K. Linde, G. Ramirez, C. D. Mulrow, A. Pauls, and W. Weidenhammer, "St. John's Wort for Depression—An Overview and Meta-analysis of Randomized Clinical Trials," *British Medical Journal* 3, no. 313 (1996): 253–58.

13. See E. U. Vorbach, W. D. Hubner, and K. H. Arnoldt, "Effectiveness and Tolerance of the Hypericum Extract LI 160 in Comparison with Imipramine: Randomized Double-Blind Study with 135 Outpatients," *Journal of Geriatric Psychiatry and Neurology* 7, suppl. 1 (1994): S19–23, and R. Bergman, J. Nuessner, and J. Demling, "Treatment of Mild to Moderate Depression: A Comparison between *Hypericum perforatum* and Amitriptyline," *Neurologie/Psychiatrie* 7 (1993): 235–40, summarized in Peter McWilliams, Mikael Nordfors, and Harold H. Bloomfield, *Hypericum and Depression* (Los Angeles: Prelude Press, 1996). These studies compared effectiveness of hypericum preparations against doses of 75 mg of imipramine, a dose most psychiatrists would probably consider barely in the usually effective range, and 30 mg of amitriptyline, a dose that is definitely subtherapeutic for most patients.

14. For a discussion of the plant origins and potent toxicity of several poisons, see Joel Hardman, Alfred Goodman Gilman, and Lee Limbird, *Goodman and Gilman's The Pharmacological Basis of Medical Therapeutics,* 9th ed. (New York: McGraw-Hill, Health Professions Division, 1996), 178–90 (strychnine and related compounds), 146–49 (amatoxins), and 149–54 (the belladonna alkaloids).

CHAPTER 10. ELECTROCONVULSIVE THERAPY

1. Emil Kraepelin, *Manic-Depressive Insanity and Paranoia,* trans. R. M. Barclay, ed. G. M. Robertson (1921; reprint, New York: Arno Press, 1976), 97.

2. C. Freeman and R. E. Kendell, "ECT I: Patients' Experiences and Attitudes," *British Journal of Psychiatry* 137 (1980): 8–16.

3. Larry Squire, Pamela Slater, and Patricia Miller, "Retrograde Amnesia and Bilateral Electroconvulsive Therapy, Long Term Follow-up," *Archives of General Psychiatry* 38 (1981): 89–95.

4. C. L. Freeman, D. Weeks, and R. E. Kendell, "ECT III: Patients Who Complain," *British Journal of Psychiatry* 137 (1980): 17–25.

5. Larry R. Squire and Pamela C. Slater, "Electroconvulsive Therapy and Complaints of Memory Dysfunction: A Prospective Three-Year Follow-up Study," *British Journal of Psychiatry* 142 (1983): 1–8.

6. American Psychiatric Association, "Practice Guidelines for the Treatment of Patients with Bipolar Disorder," *American Journal of Psychiatry* 151, suppl. (1994): 15.

7. Frederick K. Goodwin and Kay Redfield Jamison, *Manic-Depressive Illness* (New York: Oxford University Press, 1990), 661.

8. Sukdeb Mukherjee, Harold Sackeim, and David Schnur, "Electroconvulsive Therapy of Acute Manic Episodes: A Review of Fifty Years' Experience," *American Journal of Psychiatry* 151 (1994): 169–76.

9. S. Mukherjee, H. Sackeim, and C. Lee, "Unilateral ECT in the Treatment of Manic Episodes," *Convulsive Therapy* 4 (1988): 74–80.

10. Much of the work comparing the effectiveness of ECT with that of medication compares it with treatment with lithium. As studies comparing it with treatment with newer agents (such as the anticonvulsants) are done, statements about ECT's superiority to medical treatments for mania may need to be revised. However, given that the new mood stabilizers are perhaps *less* effective than lithium for depression, ECT's claims as a more predictably effective treatment for bipolar depression remain unchallenged.

11. See Mark S. George, Eric Wasserman, and Robert Post, "Transcranial Magnetic Stimulation: A Neuropsychiatric Tool for the Twenty-first Century," *Journal of Neuropsychiatry and Clinical Neurosciences* 8 (1996): 373–82.

12. Mark George, Eric Wasserman, Tim Kimbrell, John Little, Wendol Williams, Aimee Danielson, Benjamin Greenberg, Mark Hallett, and Robert Post, "Mood Improvement Following Daily Left Prefrontal Repetitive Transcranial Magnetic Stimulation in Patients with Depression: A Placebo Controlled Crossover Trial," *American Journal of Psychiatry* 154 (1997): 1752–56.

13. A. Pascual-Leone, B. Rubio, F. Pallardo, and M. D. Catala, "Beneficial Effect of Rapid-Rate Transcranial Magnetic Stimulation of the Left Dorsolateral Prefrontal Cortex in Drug-Resistant Depression," *Lancet* 348 (1996): 233–37, and Charles Epstein, Gary Figiel, William McDonald, Jody Amazon-Leece, and Linda Figiel, "Rapid Rate Transcranial Magnetic Stimulation in Young and Middle-Aged Refractory Depressed Patients," *Psychiatric Annals* 28 (1998): 36–39.

CHAPTER 11. COUNSELING AND PSYCHOTHERAPY

1. Jan Scott, "Psychotherapy for Bipolar Disorder," *British Journal of Psychiatry* 167 (1995): 581–88.

2. Nick Kanas, "Group Psychotherapy with Bipolar Patients: A Review and Synthesis," *International Journal of Group Psychotherapy* 43 (1993): 321–33.

3. L. E. Pollack, "Content Analysis of Groups for Inpatients with Bipolar Disorder," *Applied Nursing Research* 6 (1993): 19–27.

4. Many articles on this type of therapy now use the term *cognitive-behavioral therapy* to describe it. Psychologist Donald Meichenbaum has written extensively on Beck's cognitive therapy as well as on other types of therapy that use the techniques of behavioral psychology to help change thinking patterns (cognition). He is perhaps most responsible for creating the broader category of "cognitive-behavioral therapy." (See Donald Meichenbaum and Roy Cameron, "Cognitive-Behavior Therapy," in *Contemporary Behavior Therapy: Conceptional and Empirical Foundations*, ed. G. Terence Wilson and Cyril M. Franks [New York: Guilford Press, 1982], 310–37.) Although some researchers and theoreticians will describe subtle differences between the terms *cognitive therapy* and *cognitive-behavioral therapy*, they now seem to be used interchangeably by most clinical psychologists—at least they are by five out of the five psychologist colleagues of mine whom I asked about it—and by researchers as well.

5. The area of comparison studies of psychotherapy and medication in the treatment of depression can be accurately described as a hornet's nest of controversy. It's not difficult to find a study to support any possible view: superiority of medication over psychotherapy, superiority of psychotherapy over medication, and equal efficacy for both. A nicely designed and well-executed study that found cognitive therapy to be as helpful as imipramine for 107 patients with major depressive disorder is Steven Hollon, Robert DeRubeis, Mark Evans, Marlin Wiemer, Michael Garvey, William Grove, and Vincente Tuason, "Cognitive Therapy and Pharmacotherapy for Depression, Singly and in Combination," *Archives of General Psychiatry* 49 (1992): 774–81. Readers who would like to jump into the hornet's nest feet first are referred to Jacqueline Persons, Michael Thase, and Paul Crits-Chistoph, "The Role of Psychotherapy in the Treatment of Depression: Review of Two Practice Guidelines," *Archives of General Psychiatry* 53 (1996): 283–90, and to the four (yes, four) accompanying rebuttal/commentary articles in the same issue of *Archives*.

6. Beck, Rush, Shaw, and Emery, *Cognitive Therapy of Depression*, 11.

7. The linguistic purist in me wants the plural of *schema* to be *schemata* or perhaps *schemae*. But *schemas* is the plural used in cognitive-therapy literature.

8. See Jan Scott, "Cognitive Therapy of Affective Disorders: A Review," *Journal of Affective Disorders* 37 (1996): 1–11.

9. David J. Miklowitz, "Psychotherapy in Combination with Drug Treatment for Bipolar Disorder," *Journal of Clinical Psychopharmacology* 16, suppl. (1996): 56S–66S.

10. E. Frank, S. Hlastala, A. Ritenour, P. Houck, X. M. Tu, T. H. Monk, A. G. Mallinger, and D. J. Kupfer, "Inducing Lifestyle Regularity in Recovering Bipolar Disorder Patients: Results from the Maintenance Therapies in Bipolar Disorder Protocol," *Biological Psychiatry* 15 (1997): 1165–73.

11. Kay Redfield Jamison, *An Unquiet Mind* (New York: Vintage Books, 1995), 88–89.

CHAPTER 12. TREATMENT APPROACHES IN BIPOLAR DISORDER

1. The word *empirical* is derived from the Greek word *empeirikos,* which means "a doctor relying on experience alone." It also has the archaic meaning—at least I hope it's archaic—of "charlatan."

CHAPTER 13. BIPOLAR DISORDER IN CHILDREN AND ADOLESCENTS

1. Barbara Geller, Kai Sun, Betsy Zimerman, Joan Luby, Jeanne Frazier, and Marlene Williams, "Complex and Rapid-Cycling in Bipolar Children and Adolescents: A Preliminary Study," *Journal of Affective Disorders* 34 (1995): 259–68.

2. Roselind Neuman, Barbara Geller, John Rice, and Richard Todd, "Increased Prevalence and Earlier Onset of Mood Disorders among Relatives of Prepubertal versus Adult Probands," *Journal of the American Academy of Child and Adolescent Psychiatry* 36 (1997): 466–73.

3. American Academy of Child and Adolescent Psychiatry, "Practice Parameters for the Assessment and Treatment of Children and Adolescents with Bipolar Disorder," *Journal of the American Academy of Child and Adolescent Psychiatry* 36 (1997): 138–57. Studies cited on 140.

4. See Barbara Geller and Joan Luby, "Child and Adolescent Bipolar Disorder: Review of the Past Ten Years," *Journal of the American Academy of Child and Adolescent Psychiatry* 36 (1997): 1168–76.

5. Geller, Sun, Zimerman, Luby, Frazier, and Williams, "Complex and Rapid-Cycling in Bipolar Children and Adolescents: A Preliminary Study."

6. J. Biederman, S. Faraone, E. Mick, J. Wozniac, L. Chen, C. Ouellette, A. Marrs, J. Garcia, D. Mennin, and E. Lelon, "Attention-Deficit Hyperactivity Disorder and Juvenile Mania: An Overlooked Comorbidity?" *Journal of the American Academy of Child and Adolescent Psychiatry* 35 (1996): 997–1008.

7. J. Wozniak, J. Biederman, J. Mundy, D. Mennin, and S. V. Faraone, "A Pilot Family Study of Childhood-Onset Mania," *Journal of the American Academy of Child and Adolescent Psychiatry* 34 (1995): 1577–83.

8. See American Academy of Child and Adolescent Psychiatry, "Practice Parameters for the Assessment and Treatment of Children and Adolescents with Bipolar Disorder."

9. M. Strober, S. Schmidt-Lackner, R. Freeman, S. Bower, C. Lampert, and M. DeAntonio, "Recovery and Relapse in Adolescents with Bipolar Affective Illness: A Five-Year Naturalistic, Prospective Follow-up," *Journal of the American Academy of Child and Adolescent Psychiatry* 34 (1995): 724–31.

CHAPTER 14. WOMEN WITH BIPOLAR DISORDER:
SPECIAL CONSIDERATIONS

1. All three studies are described and referenced in Ellen Leibenluft, "Women with Bipolar Illness: Clinical and Research Issues," *American Journal of Psychiatry* 153 (1996): 163–73.

2. Douglas Maskall, Raymond Lam, Shala Misri, Lakshmi Yatham, and Athanasios Zis, "Seasonality of Symptoms in Women with Late Luteal Phase Dysphoric Disorder," *American Journal of Psychiatry* 154 (1997): 1436–41.

3. Leibenluft, "Women with Bipolar Illness: Clinical and Research Issues."

4. Ibid., 164.

5. Ibid., 166.

6. Victoria Hendrick, Vivien Burt, and Lori Altshuler, "Psychotropic Guidelines for Breast-Feeding Mothers," *American Journal of Psychiatry* 153 (1996): 1236–37.

CHAPTER 15. ALCOHOLISM AND DRUG ABUSE

1. D. A. Reger, M. E. Farm, and D. S. Rae, "Comorbidity of Mental Disorders with Alcohol and Other Drug Abuse: Results from the Epidemiologic Catchment Area Study," *Journal of the American Medical Association* 264 (1990): 2511–18.

2. Results quoted in Kathleen Brady and Susan Sonne, "The Relationship between Substance Abuse and Bipolar Disorder," *Journal of Clinical Psychiatry* 56, suppl. 3 (1995): 19–24.

3. Susan Sonne, Kathleen Brady, and W. Alexander Morton, "Substance Abuse and Bipolar Affective Disorder," *Journal of Nervous and Mental Disease* 182 (1994): 349–52.

4. Markus Henriksson, Hillevi Aro, Mauri Marttunnen, Martti Heikkinen, Erkki Isometsä, Kimmo Kuoppasalmi, and Jouko Lönnqvist, "Mental Disorders and Comorbidity in Suicide," *American Journal of Psychiatry* 150 (1993): 935–40.

CHAPTER 16. SEASONAL AFFECTIVE DISORDER AND CHRONOBIOLOGY

1. A. J. Lewy, H. A. Kern, N. E. Rosenthal, and T. A. Wehr, "Bright Artificial Light Treatment of a Manic-Depressive Patient with a Seasonal Mood Cycle," *American Journal of Psychiatry* 139 (1982): 1496–98.

2. Emil Kraepelin, *Manic-Depressive Insanity and Paranoia*, trans. R. M. Barclay, ed. G. M. Robertson (1921; reprint, New York: Arno Press, 1976), 139.

3. Norman E. Rosenthal, *Winter Blues: Seasonal Affective Disorder, What It Is and How to Overcome It* (New York: Guilford Press, 1993), 6.

4. Ibid., 9.

5. Curt Paul Richter, *Biological Clocks in Medicine and Psychiatry* (Springfield, Ill.: Charles C. Thomas, 1965), 3.

6. Ibid., 14–15. Emphasis added.

7. Diane Boivin, Charles Czeisler, Derk-Jan Dijk, Jeanne Duffy, Simon Folkard, David Minors, Peter Totterdell, and James Waterhouse, "Complex Interaction of the Sleep-Wake Cycle and Circadian Phase Modulates Mood in Healthy Subjects," *Archives of General Psychiatry* 54 (1997): 145–52.

8. Michael Terman, Leora Amira, Jiuan Terman, and Donald Ross, "Predictors of Response and Non-response to Light Treatment for Winter Depression," *American Journal of Psychiatry* 153 (1996): 1423–29.

9. Alexander Neumeister, Nicole Praschak-Rieder, Barbara Heßelmann, Marie-Luise Rao, Judith Glück, and Siegfried Kasper, "Effects of Tryptophan Depletion on Drug-Free Patients with Seasonal Affective Disorder during a Stable Response to Bright Light Therapy," *Archives of General Psychiatry* 54 (1997): 133–38.

10. Alan O. Kogan and Patricia Guilford, "Side Effects of Short-Term 10,000-Lux Light Therapy," *American Journal of Psychiatry* 155 (1998): 293–94.

11. Scott Campbell and Patricia Murphy, "Extraocular Circadian Phototransduction in Humans," *Science* 279 (1998): 396–99.

12. Dan A. Oren and Michael Terman, "Tweaking the Human Circadian Clock with Light," *Science* 279 (1998): 333–34.

13. A comprehensive and very readable discussion of SAD is Rosenthal, *Winter Blues.*

14. Frederick K. Goodwin and Kay Redfield Jamison, *Manic-Depressive Illness* (New York: Oxford University Press, 1990), 556–57. Chapter 19 of that volume, "Sleep and Biological Rhythms," has a comprehensive discussion of the issues presented in this chapter.

15. F. Benedetti, B. Barbini, A. Lucca, E. Campori, C. Colombo, and E. Smeraldi, "Sleep Deprivation Hastens the Antidepressant Action of Fluoxetine," *European Archives of Psychiatry and Clinical Neuroscience* 247 (1997): 100–103.

16. T. Wehr, D. Sack, and N. Rosenthal, "Sleep Reduction as a Final Common Pathway in the Genesis of Mania," *American Journal of Psychiatry* 144 (1987): 201–4.

CHAPTER 17. THE GENETICS OF BIPOLAR DISORDER

1. Emil Kraepelin, *Manic-Depressive Insanity and Paranoia,* trans. R. M. Barclay, ed. G. M. Robertson (1921; reprint, New York: Arno Press, 1976), 165.

2. For a more detailed account that includes references to the original articles, see Eliot Marshall, "Manic Depression: Highs and Lows on the Research Roller Coaster," *Science* 264 (1994): 1693–95.

3. An overview of this work is provided in Melvin McGinnis, "Recent Advances in the Genetics of Bipolar Disorder," *Psychiatric Annals* 27 (1997): 482–88.

4. Anca Ram, Françoise Guedj, Anibal Cravchik, Lee Weinstein, Qiuhe Coa, Judith Badner, Lynn Goldin, Nimrod Grisaru, Husseini Manji, Robert Belmaker, Elliot Gershon, and Pablo Gejman, "No Abnormality in the Gene for the G Protein Stimulatory α Subunit in Patients with Bipolar Disorder," *Archives of General Psychiatry* 54 (1997): 44–48.

5. See Elliot Gershon, "Genetics," in *Manic-Depressive Illness,* Frederick K. Goodwin and Kay Redfield Jamison (New York: Oxford University Press, 1990), 373–401.

6. For a very readable overview of some of these issues, see Doris Teichler Zallen, *"Does It Run in the Family?" A Consumer's Guide to DNA Testing for Genetic Disorders* (New Brunswick, N.J.: Rutgers University Press, 1997).

CHAPTER 18. BIPOLAR BIOLOGY

1. Marshall Folstein, Susan Folstein, and Paul McHugh, "Mood Disorder as a Specific Complication of Stroke," *Journal of Neurosurgery and Psychiatry* 40 (1977): 1018–20.

2. R. Robinson and T. Price, "Post-stroke Depressive Disorders: A Follow-up Study of 103 Patients," *Stroke* 13 (1982): 635–41.

3. For an in-depth discussion of the relationship between mood disorders and stroke, see Robert G. Robinson and Javier I. Travella, "Neuropsychiatry of Mood Dis-

orders," in *Neuropsychiatry*, ed. Barry S. Fogel, Randolph B. Schiffer, and Stephen M. Rao (Baltimore: Williams and Wilkins, 1996), 287–305.

4. M. Shetty and D. Lynn, "Valproate as Prophylaxis for Steroid-Induced Mood Disturbance: A Case Report," poster #51 presented at the Second International Conference on Bipolar Disorder, sponsored by the University of Pittsburgh School of Medicine, Center for Continuing Education in the Health Sciences, Pittsburgh, June 19, 1997.

5. Lori Altshuler, John Curran, Peter Hauser, Jim Mintz, Kirk Denikoff, and Robert Post, "T_2 Hyperintensities in Bipolar Disorder: Magnetic Resonance Imaging Comparison and Literature Meta-analysis," *American Journal of Psychiatry* 152 (1995): 1139–44.

6. Monte Buchsbaum, Toshiyuki Someya, Joseph Wu, Cheuk Tang, and William Bunney, "Neuroimaging Bipolar Illness with Positron Emission Tomography and Magnetic Resonance Imaging," *Psychiatric Annals* 27 (1997): 480–95.

7. Hady Shimon, Galila Agam, R. H. Belmaker, Thomas Hyde, and Joel Kleinman, "Reduced Frontal Cortex Inositol Levels in Postmortem Brain of Suicide Victims and Patients with Bipolar Disorder," *American Journal of Psychiatry* 154 (1997): 1148–50.

8. E. Fuller Torrey, Robert Rawlings, Jacqueline Ennis, Deborah Merrill, and Donn Flores, "Birth Seasonality in Bipolar Disorder, Schizophrenia, Schizoaffective Disorder, and Stillbirths," *Schizophrenia Research* 21 (1996): 141–49.

9. Robert H. Yolken, "Molecular Analysis of Brains from Individuals with Bipolar Disorder: Evidence of Viral Infections," paper presented at the Second International Conference on Bipolar Disorder, sponsored by the University of Pittsburgh School of Medicine, Center for Continuing Education in the Health Sciences, Pittsburgh, June 21, 1997.

10. Zhen Fang Fu, Jay D. Amsterdam, Moujahed Kao, Vidya Shankar, Hilary Koprowski, and Bernhard Dietzschold, "Detection of Borna Disease Virus-Reactive Antibodies from Patients with Affective Disorders by Western Immunoblot Technique," *Journal of Affective Disorders* 27 (1993): 61–68.

CHAPTER 19. BIPOLAR DISORDER AND CREATIVITY

1. Aristotle, attributed by Seneca in *Moral Essays*, "De tranquillitate animi" (On Tranquility of Mind), sec. 17, subsec. 10, quoted in *The Columbia Dictionary of Quotations* (New York: Columbia University Press, 1993; CD ROM ed., 1994).

2. Quoted in Kay Redfield Jamison, *Touched with Fire: Manic-Depressive Illness and the Artistic Temperament* (New York: Free Press, 1994), 203–5.

3. These studies are described and cited in ibid.

4. Emil Kraepelin, *Manic-Depressive Insanity and Paranoia*, trans. R. M. Barclay, ed. G. M. Robertson (1921; reprint, New York: Arno Press, 1976), 17.

5. Quoted in Jamison, *Touched with Fire*, 126.

6. Jean Cocteau, "Le coq et l'arlequin," in *Le rappel à l'ordre* (1926), quoted in *Columbia Dictionary of Quotations*, CD ROM ed.

7. These studies are cited and described in Frederick K. Goodwin and Kay Redfield Jamison, *Manic-Depressive Illness* (New York: Oxford University Press, 1990), 365–66.

CHAPTER 20. LIVING WITH BIPOLAR DISORDER

1. Emil Kraepelin, *Manic-Depressive Insanity and Paranoia,* trans. R. M. Barclay, ed. G. M. Robertson (1921; reprint, New York: Arno Press, 1976), 179–81.

2. For a complete discussion of these animal models of the kindling phenomenon, see Robert Post, "Transduction of Psychosocial Stress into the Neurobiology of Recurrent Affective Disorder," *American Journal of Psychiatry* 149 (1992): 999–1010.

3. Constance Hammen and Michael Gitlin, "Stress Reactivity in Bipolar Patients and Its Relation to Prior History of Disorder," *American Journal of Psychiatry* 154 (1997): 856–57.

4. Mario Maj, Raffaele Pirozzi, and Lorenza Magliano, "Non-response to Reinstituted Lithium Prophylaxis in Previously Responsive Bipolar Patients: Prevalence and Predictors," *American Journal of Psychiatry* 152 (1995): 1810–11. A similar study concluded that "the efficacy of lithium did not differ significantly" when it was started a second time in patients who had stopped it. But almost 13 percent of these patients needed *another* medication added to the lithium to achieve remission the second time around. (This seems to me to indicate that the lithium was *not* as effective the second time around.) See Leonardo Tondo, Ross Baldessarini, Gianfranco Floris, and Nereida Rudas, "Effectiveness of Restarting Lithium Treatment after Its Discontinuation in Bipolar I and Bipolar II Patients," *American Journal of Psychiatry* 154 (1997): 548–50.

5. Erving Goffman, *Stigma: Notes on the Management of Spoiled Identity* (Englewood Cliffs, N.J.: Prentice-Hall, 1963), 1, 2.

CHAPTER 21. PLANNING FOR EMERGENCIES

1. Frederick K. Goodwin and Kay Redfield Jamison, *Manic-Depressive Illness* (New York: Oxford University Press, 1990), 228–30.

2. See, for example, J. E. Bailey, A. L. Kellerman, G. W. Somes, J. G. Banton, F. Rivara, and N. Rushforth, "Risk Factors for Violent Death of Women in the Home," *Archives of Internal Medicine* 157 (1997): 777–82.

3. *American Heritage Dictionary of the English Language,* 3d ed. (New York: Houghton Mifflin, 1992).

CHAPTER 22. THE ROLE OF THE FAMILY

1. Kay Redfield Jamison, *An Unquiet Mind: A Memoir of Moods and Madness* (New York: Vintage Books, 1996), 120.

2. Stephen Strakowski, Susan McElroy, Paul Keck, and Scott West, "Suicidality among Patients with Mixed and Manic Bipolar Disorder," *American Journal of Psychiatry* 153 (1996): 674–76.

CHAPTER 23. LOOKING AHEAD

1. R. E. Hoffman, "Attractor Neural Networks and Psychotic Disorders," *Psychiatric Annals* 22 (1992): 119–24.

Index

heredity. *See* genetics
"humoral theory" of bipolar disorder, 61–62
hypericum, 122–23
hypersexuality, 11
hypersomnia, 21
hyperthymic temperament, 49
hypochondria, 23
hypomania, 15–17

imipramine, 71–72, 102
interpersonal and social rhythm therapy (IP/SRT), 141–42
involuntary commitment, 244–47

James, Robert, 62
Jamison, Kay Redfield, 13, 25, 142, 212
Johns Hopkins University, 40, 179, 222

kindling hypothesis, 224–25
Klonopin, 117
Kraepelin, Emil, 1, 12, 63–64
Kuhn, Roland, 71, 79, 102

Lamictal, 97–98
lamotigine, 97–98
legal issues, 245–47
Librium, 117
light therapy, 179, 185–87
lithium: discovery of therapeutic effects of, 68–70, 84–87; side effects, 90–91; therapeutic blood levels, 88–89; therapeutic mechanism of, 81–83; therapeutic profile of, 87–89
lorazepam, 117
Luvox , 104

magnetic resonance imaging (MRI), 205
major depression: *DSM* categories, 59–60; symptoms of, 18–25
major tranquilizers. *See* antipsychotic medications
mania: in children, 160–61; origin of term, 257n; stages of, 14–15; symptoms of, 9–15
"manic-depressive illness," 8, 37. *See also* bipolar disorder
"manic-depressive insanity," 12, 63
MAOIs. *See* monoamine oxidase inhibitors
maprotiline, 102
melancholia, 59, 61

mental status examination, 29
methylphenidate, 120
Meyer, Adolf, 66–67
mirtazapine, 105
mixed affective state, 15, 20, 25–27
mixed mania, 15, 20, 25–27
monoamine oxidase inhibitors (MAOIs), 105–7
mood: abnormal, 6–9; changes in bipolar I, 32; changes in bipolar II, 39; changes in cyclothymic disorder, 44; definition of, 5; diurnal variation of, 21; reactivity of, 18–19
MRI. *See* magnetic resonance imaging

Nardil, 106
National Institutes of Mental Health (NIMH), 14–15, 40, 96, 178–79
nefazodone, 105
neurogenic amines, 80
neuroleptic. *See* antipsychotic medications
neurotransmitters: definition of, 77–79; effect of antidepressants on, 80–81, 100
norepinephrine, 79–81, 100
Norpramine , 102
nortriptyline, 102
NOS ("not otherwise specified"), in *DSM*, 45–46, 58–59

olanzapine, 114

Pamelor, 102
paranoia. *See* delusional thinking
Parnate, 106
paroxetine, 104
Paul of Aegina, 62
Paxil, 104
pellagra, 65–66
pemoline, 120
personality disorders, 43–44, 57
positron emission tomography (PET), 205–6
phenelzine, 106
phenothiazine, 110
phototherapy, 179, 185–87
PMS. *See* premenstrual syndrome
postpartum mood disorders, 168–69
pregnancy, medications during, 168–69. *See also individual medications*
premenstrual syndrome (PMS), 165–67

protriptyline, 102

Prozac, 80, 104

pseudo-parkinsonism, 112

pseudo-unipolar depression, 47

psychosis, definition, 109. *See also* delusional thinking; hallucinations

psychostimulants, 119–120

psychotherapy: development of, 66–67, 134–35; "dynamic," 142–44; types of, 134–44

quetiapine, 114

rapid-cycling bipolar disorder, 50–51, 167–68

Remeron, 105

Richter, Curt P., 179–83

Risperdal, 114

risperidone, 114

Ritalin, 120

Robinson, Robert, 200–202

Rosenthal, Norman, 178

rTMS, 130–32

SAD. *See* seasonal affective disorder

schizoaffective disorder, 51–53

schizophrenia, 51–53, 67, 70, 114, 124–25, 207

Schou, Morgans, 71, 85–86, 89

Schumann, Robert, 211–12

seasonal affective disorder (SAD), 166–67, 183–87; *DSM* category, 59

second messenger system, 82–83

selective serotonin reuptake inhibitors (SSRIs), 103–5

selegiline, 106

Seranus Ephisios, 84

Seroquel, 114

serotonin, 80, 103–4, 184–85

sertraline, 104

Serzone, 105

sexual function: in depression, 22; in mania, 11; medications affecting, 104–5; psychostimulants to improve, 120

Sinequan, 102

single proton emission computed tomography (SPECT), 250

sleep, 187–90; pattern in depression, 21–22; pattern in mania, 12

sleep deprivation, to treat depression, 189–90

"soft" bipolar disorders. *See* bipolar spectrum disorders

SPECT. *See* single proton emission computed tomography

speech patterns in mania, 11

SSRIs. *See* selective serotonin reuptake inhibitors

St. John's wort, 122–23

steroids, 203–4

stigma, 230–31

stroke, 199–202

Styron, William, 19, 20, 22, 24–25

substance abuse, 170–76

substance-induced mood disorder, 60

suicide: prevention, 238–39; rates in bipolar disorder, 170, 175, 238

support groups, 137, 229–30, 249

synapse, 78–79

syphilis, 65

tardive dyskinesia (TD), 113

TCAs. *See* tricyclic antidepressants

TD. *See* tardive dyskinesia

Tegretol. *See* carbamazepine

temperament, 43–44, 47–48

T_2 hyperintensities, 205–6

thyroid function, lithium's effects on, 91

thyroid hormones, 121, 203–4

tiagabine, 99

TMS. *See* transcranial magnetic stimulation

Tofranil. *See* imipramine

topiramate, 99

transcranial magnetic stimulation (TMS), 130–32

Tranxene, 117

tranylcypromine, 106

tricyclic antidepressants (TCAs), 100–103

Valium, 117

valproate: blood levels, 94; discovery of therapeutic effects of, 92; side effects, 94–95

van Gogh, Vincent, 209–10

venlafaxine, 104

viruses, 206–8

Vivactil, 102

LIBRARY OF CONGRESS CATALOGING-IN-PUBLICATION DATA

Mondimore, Francis Mark, 1953–
    Bipolar disorder : a guide for patients and families / Francis Mark Mondimore.
       p.   cm. — (A Johns Hopkins Press health book)
    Includes bibliographical references and index.
    ISBN 0-8018-6117-9 (alk. paper). — ISBN 0-8018-6118-7 (pbk. : alk. paper)
    1. Manic-depressive illness—Popular works.   2. Affective disorders—Popular works.
I. Title. II. Series.
    [DNLM: 1. Bipolar Disorder—diagnosis popular works.   2. Bipolar Disorder—
therapy popular works.   WM 207 M741b   1999]
    RC516.M64   1999
    616.89′5—DC21
    DNLM/DLC for Library of Congress   98-41913
                                                                     CIP